Understanding

Canine
Epileptoid
Cramping
Syndrome

By Stacey Firth

The information in this book is taken from my own research and findings into CECS. It is intended for educational purposes and is not meant to replace veterinary medical treatment. Due to CECS being very similar to other conditions you must consult your vet to rule out other illnesses.

This book is for your own personal use and should not be reproduced, stored in a retrieval system, or transmitted in any form or by means, electronic, mechanical, photocopying, recording or otherwise, without the prior permission of the copyright owner. All research findings in this book was privately funded by the author.

Dedicated to Jan Gale

For all your help, support and fighting for the cause

Kes & Penny

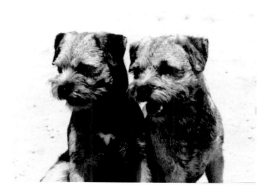

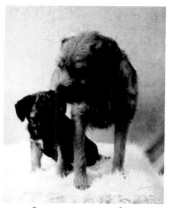

In memory of Lucy

Lucy & Josh

Contents

Introduction

Let me tell you a little bit about myself and how I got involved with CECS research.

My name is Stacey and in 2007 my first BT called Lucy suffered her first CECS episode. She was just coming up to 2 years and 8 months old. Having lived with an epileptic dog a few years before I quickly realised that this was not epilepsy. I contacted the breeder and explained what had happened. He told me that Lucy's mother suffered from a similar condition when she was in season. He suggested that I had her spayed and it would stop.

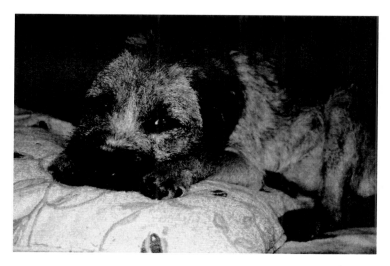

Lucy Aged 2

I searched the internet which was limited back then but I came across a lady called Jan Gale who was very helpful and showed compassion towards mine and Lucy's predicament.

Jan became involved in research regarding this condition after her beloved Kes showed signs and symptoms of what we now call CECS. She wondered whether the condition was hereditary due to a little mate, Penny, showing the same signs. After speaking to her vet and her own research she soon came to realise that diet may be a key to managing the symptoms.

She explained about the disorder CECS and she gave me valuable advice which I put into practice.

After speaking to various vets and organisations no-one had any answers to my questions but it was apparent there was a health problem with Border Terriers not just in England but Europe and worldwide too. Quite a lot of vets had not heard of this condition and most of them diagnosed that Lucy was suffering from a form of epilepsy.

As far as I could see there was limited research into this condition and a lack of knowledge.

I decided to seek the answers not just to my questions but for other owners who were living with a CECS sufferer.

In order to understand and develop my knowledge and understanding how the canine body worked. I undertook an educational course in Canine Development in America. To further my understanding in CECS I also undertook courses and gained qualifications in canine nutrition, understanding the major organs as well as the workings of the digestive system.

I spent another 3 years gaining the knowledge and qualifications needed to research, evaluate and find a way to manage this condition using herbal supplements as well as Flower remedies and the holistic approach to canine illnesses.

With most human illness, we rely on the patient being able to explain how they feel and where the problem is coming from. Unfortunately, a dog cannot tell us so we have to rely on the owner or we need to read and understand the dog's signals.

With this in mind, I returned to college and gained the qualification in Canine Psychology and Canine awareness.

Finally, in 2012 I began the research tests on CECS sufferers which gave me knowledge regarding the condition and the stages before an episode.

My research led me to a certain type of protein which makes up the DNA structure of a Border Terrier. The Border Terrier is still a new breed compared to other breeds of dogs which have been around for hundreds of years. Bred as a fox and vermin hunter, the Border Terrier shares ancestry with the Dandie Dinmont Terrier and the Bedlington Terrier. These two breeds do have their own health problems which can be hereditary and passed down through the Bedlington line but research has shown that only a small percentage of Border Terriers have shown symptoms of those breeds illnesses.

The environment that we live in today has changed the way people live, eat and sleep.

Technology has taken over and with the internet comes social media, google and much more information about what we should feed and care for our dogs. We are offered advice which sometimes is misleading.

Our lifestyles and our environment are changing and what people fail to realise it's having an impact on our dog's health.

As little as 30 years ago a small terrier would live on average18 years.

20 years ago, it declined to 15 years on average.

Today its dropped to a frightening 12 -14 years of age.

Today we see more cars on the road and ongoing environmental issues. Small dogs are more at risk than other breeds due to the level that exhaust fumes are expelled. Living in the urban belt your dog is more at risk from allergies, breathing problems, major organ disease, cataracts and tumours. There has been an increase in brain tumours and nasal tumours.

The same is happening within the pet food market. Most companies are always trying to find ways to decrease out goings and increase their customer base. This can be done with replacing natural products like meat protein and vital nutrients with a chemical substitute. They also want to please the owners as well as the dog in making you think that their product is vital to keep your dog healthy. Most processed pet foods main ingredient is a filler. This can be rice, grains, potato and other products which do not contain any nutritional value whatsoever.

Well a chain reaction is at work. Taken into account the environmental issue's combined with the ever-increasing processed food manufacturing your dog is at risk even more today than that is was 10 years ago.

One of the most important thing an animal needs is a fully functioning immune system. If this fails by 5% the affects it has on your dog can be costly and even life threatening.

With this in mind the main function to keeping your dog healthy is 'the immune system'. If this breaks down the liver, the pancreas and the kidney's start to fail at removing everyday toxins. This can result in increased allergies, whether they are diet or external skin related.

Questions and answers based on my own research.

I have tried to keep the answers readable and understandable for the pet owner.

What is Canine Epileptoid Cramping Syndrome?

- **Canine:** Dog

- **Epileptoid:** Having the character of or resembling epilepsy but is not epilepsy

- **Cramping:** Sudden and painful involuntary contractions of the muscles

- **Syndrome:** A collection of signs & symptoms that appear together to form a collection

Why was it called Spikes disease?

Spike was one of the first dogs to be recognised with the disorder.

What are the symptoms of CECS?

My research found that most symptoms of CECS are triggered related.

These are some of my findings:

- Sickness

- Yellow & white bile regurgitation

- Abdominal noise

- Trembling

- Disorientation

- Slow posturing

- Involuntary muscle contractions

- Complete collapse

- Unable to stand

- Dizziness

What are the triggers?

Any of these triggers can result in mild to more severe forms of a CECS episode. These are just a few triggers I have found while researching CECS.

- Heat

- Cold

- Diet (Gluten & no gluten)

- Stress

- Fear

- Pain

- Depression

- Vaccinations & Boosters including Kennel cough

- Metal contamination

- Hormonal

- Salts

- Sugars

- Artificial colourings & preservatives

- Liver & kidney disorders

- Inflamed pancreas

- Exercise

- Excitement

- Chemicals (Flea treatments, wormers, conventional medicines)

*Data collected from CECS Facebook group. Owners reported known triggers which affected their dog. Beef, raw hide, heat, worming products, fish, stress, grains, flea treatments, meat, excitement, gluten, high protein, empty tummies, lamb, fatty meats, changes in the house, noise, hot weather, hormone related, turkey, chicken, liver, dry processed food, grass eating, pig's ears, shock, cheese, cooked ham, fireworks, thunderstorms, anxiety, dreaming, change of routine, vaccinations and boosters, cold weather, wheat, underweight, overweight.

Why doesn't my dog show all the Symptoms?

My research findings have brought me to the conclusion that there are three stages to CECS. It all depends on what stage they are at, the known triggers and how the condition manifest itself. (See theory on stages)

My theory based on the research I have obtained over the last few years.

Stage one

- Digestion – The correct diet for the needs of the dog. Whether the outside temp is affecting the inner temp when the digestive process takes place. Whether the dog is getting the correct protein, nutrients and vitamins from their diet. Whether the body is finding it difficult to digest sugars, salt and vital minerals. The immune system may not be working correctly and is finding it hard to remove toxins and fight off bacteria. Too much gas is being produced after eating a meal. Toxins are present in your dog's diet, whether it is processed food or a raw diet. The body itself can produce toxins while the digestion process is taking place.

If any of the above factors are encountered it can result in cramping of the stomach, swelling of the abdomen, popping noise and slight movement of the belly which can cause trembling or slight shaking. A dog can be picky when it comes to food due to pain it may be experiencing after eating a meal so it's reluctant to eat the next one. Regurgitation of white or yellow bile may be present up to 8 hours after your dog has eaten. They show an interest in eating of grass or other green plants in and around your garden. If your dog is at stage one my research has found that most dogs can go about their daily routines and it doesn't always seem to affect them.

Stage one can be confused with other illnesses and diseases. Dogs can tremble after eating due to many reasons, the portion was too large, the food was not their usual diet, feeling sick due to over production of bile and the feeling of sickness due to the speed the dog may have eaten.

We need to try and identify and rule out any other contributing factors which may also be causing the above symptoms.

A breakdown in the digestion process can cause the above symptoms. Eating contaminated toxins whether present in their diet or may have been digested by other means such as accidental poisoning.

Early stages of pancreatitis, liver and kidney problems. Allergy towards one or more ingredient in their diet (gluten, wheat, soy, artificial proteins and many other products which can cause an intolerance).

Gall bladder, pancreas and bile communication breakdown.

Diabetes, Cushing's, UTI and many more conditions which our dogs may be suffering from.

If this stage happens once every so often I would suggest that you monitor the situation and take note of what you have fed your dog (the ingredient), when and how long these symptoms have lasted.

We need to take into account whether their diet is correct one for their needs. We need to look at chemicals which may be entering your dog's digestive system, whether your dog is in good health and the immune system is working correctly. We also need to take into account any environmental factors which may be having an impact on the dog as a whole.

Stage two

- Hepatic breakdown

Due to the digestion issue accompanied with the trigger, I believe that the liver and the bile production begins to overwork to try to compensate for the breakdown of the digestion process. It's at this stage that I believe toxins and gases are leaked into the blood supply.

Your dog can show symptoms of severe trembling, exaggerated stretching, staggering, unable to move fast, lip smacking, sickness, grass eating and showing no interest in their daily routine. If you conducted a liver function test the results may show elevated Alanine transaminase. ALT is an enzyme that helps break down proteins and is found mainly in the liver.

Alkaline phosphatase (ALP) test. ALP is an enzyme you have in your liver, bile ducts, and bone, again this could be elevated in some cases.

This tells us that the liver is not functioning to its full capacity. Usually, if the readings are high along with other symptoms which are not present at stage two CECS could indicate liver disease or a related issue with the pancreas. Usually, the vet will conduct another test a few days later to find whether the levels have decreased. If not, they will do more tests to verify the cause of the issue.

My research has shown that in most cases where CECS is apparent that the levels have returned to normal the next day or even a few hours after the stage two process.

Again, I must point out at this stage that veterinary help is needed to eliminate other disease or illness. The above symptoms could indicate a more life threating issue which needs resolving urgently. Your vet may want to take a bile test to rule out Hepatic microvascular dysplasia. They may also check for a liver shunt and other illnesses and diseases.

Stage three

- Neurological

This is what I call a true episode. At this stage, CECS takes on a neurological form due to the breakdown of the blood brain barrier. It is there to filter and remove any toxins or waste which could impede the central nervous system. At stage three your dog may completely collapse and is unable to stand but is conscious. They may show signs of cramping in his hind legs, arching of the back which may alleviate any stomach cramps. Front legs can be fully stretched out to their capacity, they can empty their bladder or bowels due to the build-up of any gases in the intestines. They may drool with saliva, but not froth. They appear to be disorientated and show that they need reassurance from an owner. The episodes can last from 20 secs to a full 35 mins (taken from the research I conducted in 2014). An episode can be reoccurring and can be mild to severe.

Medication can be used to alleviate cramps; the common ones are Diazepam or Clorazepate. I don't usually suggest these drugs because again you are forcing chemicals into their system when some don't really need them. This has to be your choice and, in some cases, help but in other cases they are not needed. Usually, a dog will return to normal after the episode has passed, some owners have reported their dog can be very tired after an episode.

It's at this stage that a diagnosis is needed to rule out epilepsy.

The vet may run further tests such as an electroencephalogram (EEG) or magnetic resonance imaging (MRI). Your dog is relying on you as an owner to convey what happened exactly to the vet. Due to CECS being such a young illness some vets are unaware of this condition and treat your dogs for epilepsy.

How can I tell the difference between Epilepsy, CECS or another kind of seizure?

Seizures and episodes can strike at any time. Understanding why they have happened and what kind of seizure can be a little bit harder to determine except for eliminating characteristic normally associated with epilepsy and other medical condition.

How CECS episodes differ to an epileptic seizure is that your dog will be conscious through-out the episode, they will be aware of their surroundings and don't usually lose bladder or bowel control. With epilepsy a dog tends to chatter its jaw and shake uncontrollably and will not respond to your voice or its surroundings.

Working with your vet they can determine what may have caused a seizure i.e. brain tumour, infections, brain trauma, poisoning, low blood sugar, hypothyroidism. Your veterinarian can discuss a variety of diagnostic tests such as blood work, x-rays, CT scan, MRI, Spinal fluid tap. These tests are essential to rule out other illnesses before diagnosing your dog with CECS.

Which breeds does it affect?

Currently, we know through research that CECS mainly affects Border Terriers but other breeds have reported similar symptoms and are being investigated.

Is every Border terrier affected?

No, not all Border Terriers are affected by CECS. Research is being conducted to try to identify a faulty gene which may be responsible for this illness.

How do you know if an animal is a carrier or likely to become affected?

There is currently no test to identify individuals who may develop the condition when older. It is recommended not to purchase puppies from affected parents or from parents which have previously produced affected offspring. It seems likely that carrier animals exist, that is, that some animals may carry the abnormal gene without developing the disease themselves. † It is thought that this disease has a genetic basis because of its occurrence in certain bloodlines of this breed and it has been suggested that it may be due to an autosomal recessive gene back in 2005. However, this has not been confirmed and the mode of inheritance is not currently known.

†Leitchty M and Blake K (2005) Canine epileptoid cramping, a syndrome in border terriers. National Border Terrier Specialty CECS Seminar. 6th June 2005

What has changed in the development of Border Terriers for this condition to exist?

It is common knowledge that most breeds suffer from certain conditions which effect their health. These are some of the known illnesses or diseases in some other breeds.

- **Siberian Husky: Autoimmune Disorders**
- **Bulldog: Respiratory Problems**
- **Pug: Eye Problems**
- **German Shepherd: Hip Dysplasia**
- **Labrador Retriever: Obesity**
- **Beagle: Epilepsy**
- **Shih Tzu: Wobbly Kneecaps**
- **Boxer: Cancer**
- **Dachshund: Back Problems**
- **Doberman Pinscher: Heart Condition**
- **Cocker Spaniel: Ear Infections**
- **Yorkshire Terrier: Portosystemic Shunt**
- **Poodle: Glaucoma**
- **Rottweiler: Joint Problems**
- **Miniature Schnauzer: Diabetes**
- **Chihuahua: Collapsing Trachea**
- **Great Dane: Bloat**
- **Maltese: Little White Shaker Syndrome**
- **Boston Terrier: Cherry Eye**
- **French Bulldog: Breathing Problems**
- **Cavalier King Charles Spaniel: Mitral Valve Disease**

The history of the Border Terrier

Most breeds of dogs have been around for hundreds of years. The Border Terrier is still a young breed compared to some other breeds and CECS could have been a heredity illness waiting to happen. As the breed ages, new defects are now coming to light and unfortunately it could be down to the natural development of the breed or it could be due to man's invention of developing a perfect border terrier.

I have found documentation from 100 years ago that shows that the breed has changed since over the last 110 years.

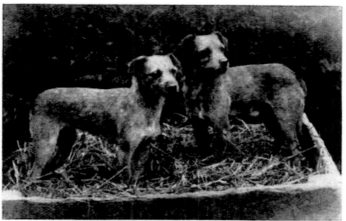

Flint and Fury about 1900

Flint and Fury were two of the very first Border Terriers. Flint, the dog on the right, was whelped in 1894 by Jacob Robson's Rock out of Tom Robson's Rat. Fury, the bitch on the left, was sired by Flint and whelped in 1898 out of bitch by the name of Vene.

The famous terrier Flint, weighing 12 pounds, could bolt foxes out of holes which had hitherto been considered impossible places. They stand 14 inches high and are narrow in front, not more than 15 in. round the girth.

Not many Border Terriers look like that today and are very rarely used in the field due to the breed growing in size and being less tolerant to taking orders.

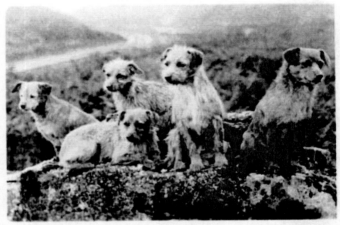

1915 A group of Willie Barton's early Border Terriers Left to Right: Bess I, Willie Barton's first Border, born 1900, bred by Mr. J.T. Dodd, of Riccarton; Viper (lying) and Venom, by Nailer ex Venus; Piper, also ex Venus; and Venus. Piper was grandsire of Ch Liddesdale Bess, dam of Dubh Glas.

Borders in those earlier days were somewhat different from the current show version. The earlier Border, who was bred for work rather than exhibition, was certainly smaller than many borders we see winning today, who can reach 16-18" at the withers and weigh 20-24 pounds.

Could CECS be related to a liver shunt?

I have found through my research that only a few Border Terriers who have CECS in fact have a liver shunt. The symptoms are very similar and a liver shunt can cause mild tremors to full blown seizures, but not in all cases. The theory behind a liver shunt is very similar to my findings that CECS is a combination of digestive issues and toxic substances entering the brain through the blood brain barrier.

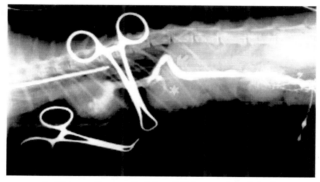

In this radiograph, blood (shown in white)
flows through a shunt (arrow) bypassing
the liver (star).

One of the jobs of the liver is to ensure that only the good stuff from the food we eat gets into the body. Dogs are notorious for eating disgusting things, such as the mouldy cheese out of the garbage, and their liver is responsible for keeping toxins from affecting the body. In addition, the action of bacteria in the intestines on food can produce toxic by-products which the liver deals with. All the blood coming from the intestines goes through the liver first, where it is cleansed of toxins before going around the rest of the body. When an embryo is safe in the mother's womb, the mother's liver takes care of that job, and the embryo doesn't need to worry about it. As a result, the blood from the intestines bypasses the liver in the embryo through a separate vessel called a shunt. When the pup is born, however, the liver needs to switch gears and start doing its job of cleaning the blood from the intestines, therefore the shunt closes down and blood is run through the liver to be cleansed before it gets to the brain.

If the shunt fails to shut down like it should, then blood will continue to bypass the liver. A shunt that is present from birth is called a congenital shunt. The liver then doesn't get a chance to remove the bad stuff until it's already circulating around the body. Many of the toxins that the liver would normally clean up can affect the brain, and seizures can be one of the effects.

Shunts can also be acquired later in life. If the liver is diseased, blood may have a hard time flowing through the sick liver, leading to a back-pressure in the vessels coming from the intestines. The result is the same as the congenital shunt; blood bypasses the liver and toxins affect the brain.

Both because liver problems can cause seizures and because many of the medications used to treat epilepsy can injure the liver, we recommend liver function tests as part of the initial work-up and as part of the regular check-ups. The liver enzyme tests which are part of a routine chemistry profile may not be adequate to detect liver shunts and liver function tests, such as bile acids or ammonia, are necessary.

Does diet make a difference?

When choosing a diet for your dog whether they suffer from CECS or any other illness you need to take into consideration the environment which it lives in, food intolerance, allergies, weight, health and the dog's needs in general. Each dog needs a diet which is tailor made to suit them. A diet for one dog may not be suitable for another.

Some owners believe that a gluten free, low protein or a reduced fat diet has lessened the number of episodes their dog has had. In some instances, it has not made any difference to their dog and in others, they have reported an increase in colitis bouts.

Why do vets and some people suggest a gluten free diet or a low protein diet?

When CECS was first researched back in the 1970's early 80's, it was thought that CECS was brought on by a high protein diet or gluten products. It was first suggested by the earlier sufferers that they had seen a result in reducing the digestive issues and the number of episodes that their dogs were experiencing. Most of the dogs at the time were related through parentage and they may have had a gluten intolerance. Due to the lack of recent research and awareness owners and vets can only access information which can be unreliable from the internet and social media. These two diets can help some dogs but not all and with a small percentage can, in fact, harm your dog.

My research has shown that a percentage of border terriers suffer from a gluten intolerance and this can be confused with CECS.

Veterinary neurologist Mark Lowrie, has identified a new way to diagnose this problem which is most commonly known as paroxysmal gluten-sensitive dyskinesia (PGSD). Mark and his team have pioneered the use of serological markers to prove their diagnostic utility PGSD in Border terriers.

†Further information about Mark Lowrie's research can be found at
http://onlinelibrary.wiley.com/doi/10.1111/jvim.15038/pdf

Is my dog in pain when having an episode?

It's very hard to say whether they are in pain or not. What I have found out when researching CECS is every dog is different while having an episode. My first dog Lucy acted as though she was in pain while Josh appears to be distressed due to uncontrollable muscle jerks and stretching. Neither of mine has ever cried out in pain but they do show signs of being in distress. If I am correct and my theory is right that CECS is a combination of digestion problems, organs not being able to filter the toxins and due to the infiltration of toxic gases, becomes a neurology problem resulting in disorientation, involuntary muscle movement and uncontrollable nerve twitches throughout the body. If that is the case your dog may be feeling the way we would feel when we are drunk or taking certain drugs. CECS looks very distressing and everyone describes their dog's episodes differently. I have found that reassuring the dog and making sure they are safe helps the episode pass more quickly. If the muscles were under an incredible amount of pain you would find that a dog would not be able to stand up and run around 10 mins after an episode.

My research has led me to believe that CECS presents its self as a neurological problem that begins in the digestion process and how their digestive system deals with the chemical reaction while extracting and processing vitamins, nutrients and eliminating toxins.

Another illness which presents itself similar to CECS is Parkinson's disease. A study has been published recently regarding Parkinson's and it is the strongest evidence yet that Parkinson's begins in the gut and not the brain. The findings suggest that that the disease is triggered by bacteria that live in the digestive tract and it causes a build-up of a protein called alpha-synuclein within the brain.

Another similar illness to CECS is Encephalitis. This is where a virus and toxins can enter the brain via the blood brain barrier. Taking both conditions and combining my research I believe that there is a breakdown of the digestive process which allows toxins, unfriendly proteins, and bacteria to flow into the blood stream, vital organ and eventually into the brain causing a full blown CECS episode.

What you feed your dog is essential to its health and well-being. A dog can live on a very basic diet but eventually, their health will start to decline.

Whether you choose a raw, processed or a home-cooked diet there are pitfalls to all pet food diets.

To understand the process of digestion we need to look at proteins which are an important element which is vital to our dog's health.

What are proteins?

Proteins are vital component for life. Protein is an important substance found in every cell in the human body. In fact, except for water, protein is the most abundant substance in your body.

Proteins are made up of hundreds or thousands of smaller units called amino acids, which are attached to one another in long chains. There are 20 different types of amino acids that can be combined to make a protein.

Why do dogs need protein?

- **Energy**   If dogs consume more protein than they need for body tissue maintenance and other necessary functions, their body will use it for energy. If it is not needed due to sufficient intake of other energy sources such as carbohydrates, the protein will be used to create fat and becomes part of fat cells.

- **Hormones**   Protein is involved in the creation of some hormones. These substances help control body functions that involve the interaction of several organs. Insulin, a small protein, is an example of a hormone that regulates blood sugar. It involves the interaction of organs such as the pancreas and the liver. Secretin, is another example of a protein hormone. This substance assists in the digestive process by stimulating the pancreas and the intestine to create necessary digestive juices.

- **Enzymes** These are proteins that increase the rate of chemical reactions in the body. In fact, most of the necessary chemical reactions in the body would not efficiently proceed without enzymes. For example, one type of enzyme functions as an aid in digesting large protein, carbohydrate and fat molecules into smaller molecules, while another assists the creation of DNA

- **Transportation and Storage of Molecules** Protein is a major element in transportation of certain molecules. For example, haemoglobin is a protein that transports oxygen throughout the body. Protein is also sometimes used to store certain molecules. Ferritin is an example of a protein that combines with iron for storage in the liver.

- **Antibodies** Protein forms antibodies that help prevent infection, illness and disease. These proteins identify and assist in destroying antigens such as bacteria and viruses. They often work in conjunction with the other immune system cells. For example, these antibodies identify and then surround antigens in order to keep them contained until they can be destroyed by white blood cells.

Protein is very important for our dogs. If you reduce or stop all proteins it may be good in the short term but eventually, your dog may start suffering in other ways health wise if they are not getting enough protein.

What proteins are added to pet food and how do they affect our dogs?

Some owners of CECS sufferers suggest a low protein diet to help stop triggers of CECS in their pets. My research has concluded that this may not be the answer for all CECS sufferers. Protein is broken down into two categories; vegetable/Plant protein and animal protein. I have found that vegetable protein is more of a concern than protein which comes from meat. Most pet food manufacturers do not state whether the protein found in their products are animal or vegetable based. Vegetable protein (usually soy products) is a cheap and easy way to boost the protein level in your dog's diet. This type of protein can cause some dogs to have extreme stomach cramps and can result in untreatable skin allergies in others.

Vegetable/Plant protein can be bad.

Usually it is sourced from the soya bean which recently has shown can cause severe stomach and bowel cramps as well as seizure's in dogs. It is one of the main culprits behind bloat in some dogs and can also cause hyperactivity in others. Soy can be commonly listed as soya, vegetable broth, textured vegetable protein, TVP (textured vegetable protein) or TSP (textured soy protein).

Soya can cause health problems in dogs as well as humans. The soy bean contains large quantities of natural toxins or anti-nutrients. It has a potent enzyme that blocks the actions of trypsin and other enzymes needed for protein digestion. These inhibitors are tightly folded proteins that can cause serious gastric distress; reduce protein digestion and chronic deficiencies in amino acid uptake. Diets high in trypsin inhibitors can cause enlargements and pathological conditions of the pancreas, including cancer. Soybean also contains a hemagglutinin (a clot-promoting substance that causes red blood cells to clump together). This can cause high levels of enzymes in the liver which could result in not being able to digest fats correctly.

To process soya, they need to extract the oil by fermenting the product. This is achieved by using a mold cultures and other substances that radically alter its biochemistry which makes amino acids. Processing starts by cleaning the soy bean using bleach. It is then degummed and deodorised and is crushed into flakes. It is then mixed with a petroleum-based hexane solvent to extract the soy oil for human consumption. Flake waste is then toasted and ground down and it is sold to pet food manufacturers. Soy beans and other related products can be found in most dry, wet, semi-moist and canned dog food. I have also found soy in top selling brands of dog food as well as prescription foods.

The major mineral components of soya beans are potassium, sodium, calcium, magnesium, sulphur and phosphorus. Mineral content can vary widely due to both the type of soil and growing conditions for the soybean.

Another source of protein is gluten which is found in wheat, barley, bran, bleached flour, dextrin, rye and spelt to name a few (Rice is excluded from this list as it's gluten free). Quite a number of dogs are intolerant to gluten so they need a tailored diet to suit their needs. Common illness associated with gluten is coeliac disease and gluten sensitivity.

Meat protein is good

Meat protein is easily digested by the gut; it causes fewer gases so not to overstretch the stomach. It is a very efficient way of delivering protein which is needed for a dog's development. Because animals have the same components, eating animal tissue is an easy way to get this necessary nutrient. Meat protein is made up of amino acids. Amino acids help build cells and repairs tissue, form antibodies and carry oxygen throughout the body. Vital minerals found in meat protein are Potassium, phosphorus, calcium magnesium, iron, sodium, zinc, manganese, copper and selenium. Vital vitamins in meat are vitamin B1 (thiamine), Vitamin B2 (riboflavin), Niacin, pantothenic acid, vitamin B6, folate vitamin B12, vitamin E, vitamin K and vitamin D.

Meat protein is the better option when considering a diet for any dog whether it is a CECS sufferer or a not.

So, as you can see protein intake is vital in a dog's diet.

Each dog whether they suffer from CECS, colitis, allergies, pancreatitis, kidney or liver conditions needs the correct protein so it helps the body restore any proteins which have been used for development.

The digestive process explained:

Digestive System Organs:

- stomach
- pancreas
- liver
- kidney's
- gall bladder
- small intestine
- large intestine
- colon

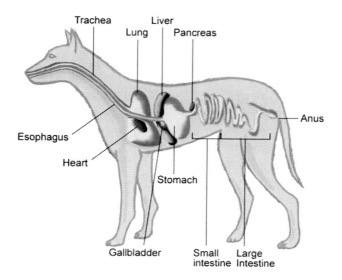

Dog digestion begins in the mouth, unlike humans the dog's salvia do not contain any enzymes to break down the food. Instead the saliva contains an enzyme which lubricates the food and kills any bacteria before it reaches the digestive system.

Unlike human's, dogs do not need to chew their food before it goes down the throat but it must be the right size and amount to fit. If not, the dog will simply throw it back up. Your dog is not being sick it's just the way the dogs body tells the dog to try again. If your dog regurgitates its food within 30 mins it is quite ok to let your dog eat what it brings up.

A dog's stomach has the ability to breakdown most of the food due to the acid. It can breakdown larger pieces of meat and bone. Food is kept in the stomach for a longer period of time. This is the reason why a dog can live with only being fed once or twice a day. They feel fuller a lot longer than a human.

Food gets broken down into a simple form that can be absorbed and used by the body in a process called "digestion." In mammals, this process takes place in the digestive or alimentary tract, often simply called the "gut." This is a hollow tube that the food passes through and is acted upon by acids and enzymes from organs, like the stomach and small intestine, which discharge into the tube. These digestive enzymes speed up the process of hydrolysis, by which food is broken down.

The three major classes of nutrients that need to be digested are carbohydrates, protein, and fat. Other nutrients (minerals, vitamins, and water) are absorbed in more or less the same form as they are found in food. But they may need to be released from proteins, fats, or carbohydrates before they can be absorbed.

It then moves onto the small intestine. More enzymes from the intestinal wall and the pancreas are added to the chyme. The pancreas is one of the major glands of the body and has two functions: releasing digestive enzymes into the gut and releasing hormones into the blood.

Pancreatic juice also contains sodium bicarbonate, which neutralizes the acidic chyme arriving in the duodenum, and provides an alkaline environment for optimum functioning of pancreatic and intestinal enzymes. These enzymes include proteases (for continued protein digestion), amylase (for carbohydrate digestion), and lipase (for fat digestion).

The regulation of pancreatic juice release is largely controlled by two hormones, secretin and pancreozymin, more commonly known as cholecystokinin. These are secreted from cells in the wall of the small intestine. Another important function of the pancreas is to secrete the hormone insulin into the bloodstream to control blood sugar levels.

44

The role of major organs

The liver is the other major organ associated with the small intestine. Bile is produced continuously in the liver, stored in the gall bladder, and passed into the gut through the bile duct when it's needed. Bile contains salts that act like detergents by turning fat into tiny globules that can then be processed by the lipase enzymes in pancreatic juice. The pigments in bile give faeces their characteristic colour.

One of the jobs of the liver is to ensure that no toxins are absorbed and only essential nutrients and vitamins are absorbed. In addition, the action of bacteria in the intestines on food can produce toxic by-products which the liver deals with. All the blood coming from the intestines goes through the liver first, where it is cleansed of toxins before going around the rest of the body.

The digestion of food is completed in the small intestine, and once the food has been broken down to its simplest form, it can be absorbed across the wall of the intestine and into the blood. The end products of digestion are carried to the liver, where they are metabolized. Fat is absorbed into the lymph vessels and is later transferred to the bloodstream.

The small intestines are very long, and absorption takes place along its entire length. Folds and finger-like projections, villi, in the lining of the intestinal wall dramatically increase the surface area for absorption.

By the time the food that have been eaten reaches the large intestine, most of the nutrients have been digested and absorbed. In this part of the gut, water is absorbed, and some fermentation of dietary fibre by bacteria takes place. This process is responsible for the production of gas, often associated with flatulence.

Faeces are around 60–70% water, and the rest is made up of undigested food, dead bacteria, and some inorganic material.

As you can see the digestion process is very complexed and it only needs a slight malfunction for things to go wrong.

One of those things can be the immune system. A good diet with the correct nutrients and vitamins will fuel the immune system and keep the body running correctly.

If the dog digestive system is malfunctioning, the immune system will even reject essential proteins unless they are first broken down by the digestive system into their primary, non-antigenic building blocks.

One thing many of us don't know is a dog on the same dog food for years will develop health problems beginning with digestion because his body is just plain worn out from trying to convert highly processed food. In that case, changing from one brand to another won't help unless it's a vast improvement or an easily digestible diet. This is one of the main reasons that vets keep prescription foods in stock. They are supposed to be tailored to suit the needs of the dog with renal problems. This is not the answer for every dog and as mentioned what is good for one dog may not be good for another. In some cases, this can cause other problems within the digestion process.

One diet for all?

All dogs are different when it comes to health and development. A small breed such as a border terrier will develop a lot sooner than a larger breed like a Great Dane. It is suggested that a smaller dog will reach its adult life by 10-month-old. That's when the body has matured and developed. A larger breed can take up to 18 months to reach the same stage.

As you can see every dog is different and each dog needs a diet which suits the needs of that particular dog.

Some vets find it difficult to suggest a suitable diet for your dog due to them not being knowledgeable in animal nutrition and the needs of that individual dog. Usually you will find that pet shops are more likely to give a valuable and knowledgeable advice on which diet are correct for your dog's needs.

If your dog suffers from digestive issue's or CECS a diet with low filler ingredient is advised.

Why do pet food manufactures add fillers to dog food?

The majority of pet food is made up of what I refer to as fillers. Fillers are the cheapest way to give bulk to the pet food with very little nutrition which the body can use. Whether you feed a dry or a wet diet they still contain bulk fillers.

Fillers can be made up from grains, cereals, rice, potato etc. If you took out the fillers you would be left with the nutritional food which your dog needs so its body can function. When dogs have food allergies whether it is digestion or skin related the main cause is due to the ingredients in the filler and not the nutritional content. Fillers usually produce gases while being digested and is one of the major causes in of bloat in dogs. The gases can cause a twisted bowel or make your dog feel uncomfortable. Stomach noises are often heard when there is a build-up of gas and the dog may look bloated and may find it hard to get comfortable.

I researched this with 2 average sized Border Terriers. We gave one a well-known and widely used brand of dog food and we gave another a home cooked meal made up from nutritional foods only. They were given exactly the same amount of food 225 grams per day. Within the first few days we noticed a big change in toilet habits from both dogs. The one on the branded dog food increased how many times it went to the toilet and the quantity expelled, it also suffered from flatulence. It was noticed that the dogs coat and breath smelled more than usual on this diet. The one on the home cooked diet reduced how many times it went to the toilet and what it expelled was greatly reduced and there were no signs of bad breath or smells coming from the coat. Both dogs weight was maintained while they were on this diet.

So, the overall outcome with fillers is why add large amounts to your dog's diet when they are not needed. The main reason is profit. The bigger the bag on the shelf the more value for money you think you are getting. When you walk out with a 15-kilo sack of dog food, just remember 70% of that is not needed, it will be expelled without any nutritional value what so ever and could be causing a build-up of trapped gasses which can cause digestion problems.

Is there a cure for CECS?

Currently there is no cure for CECS but the Animal Health Trust are storing DNA from fit and healthy Border terriers as well as CECS and other conditions which affect the breed. Eventually when they have enough samples and a DNA profile will be taken from each candidate and hopefully they will find a DNA marker which will be helpful with future Border terriers health issues.

I have two CECS sufferers, Josh who is 11 and Rusty who is 3 years old. They both have suffered from all three stages of CECS. Josh in particular has suffered from this condition for approx. 7 years. It has taken at least 3 years to find the cause, a suitable diet for his needs and a way of reducing the number of episodes and the severity of them through added supplements and flower remedies. I have not found a cure but I have found a way to manage this condition for Josh and Rusty as well as other dogs who were part of the research which I conducted a few years ago.

Is there anything I can add to my dog's food without changing their diet?

Bearing in mind the above factors I have been able to come up with a suitable supplement which can help relieve some of the symptoms of CECS. It helps by making sure your dog digestive system is extracting all the right vitamins and minerals from their diet and eliminating any toxic gases which are processed while digesting their food.

I have found in most cases that dogs that have been on the supplement have fewer episodes and if they have had them they are less severe.

What's in the Hands & Paws supplement and how does it help?

It is blend made up from chicory Inulin, a prebiotic, a live yeast probiotic, chickweed, milled linseed & dandelion root in a powder form which is sprinkled on their food.

How does the supplement work?

The live yeast helps lines the gut wall and acts as a barrier against harmful bacteria which can seep into the organs and blood supply. It works by helping to improve the uptake of vitamins, minerals, amino acids and enzymes which the body needs to function correctly. It helps eliminate toxic gases which may be produced within the digestive system. Your dog's core temperature can differ from the environmental temperature. If this happens more toxic gases are produced so heat could be a trigger for CECS sufferers without the owner realising it digestion issue's.

The chickweed contains natural vital vitamins which your dog may miss out on due to a digestive problem. The milled linseed adds natural oil to your dog's coat and skin so keeping it healthy and it also lubricates the stomach and the bowel. The dandelion root encourages your dog to eat where loss of appetite is present. It helps to settle an upset stomach, gas, muscle aches and skin conditions. It also increases the urine production so toxins are removed more regular than normal.

These products all complement each other and are vital for your dog's health. They work together and as a result they restore and maintain the immune system. It also helps stabilise stomach acids and reduces the amount of bile which is being produced. The reduction in bile helps with any reflux acid or regurgitation of yellow or white bile which can be associated with CECS.

Does having your dog neutered help reduce the symptoms?

My research has found that some CECS sufferers have reduced the number of episodes when the trigger is hormone based or due to excitement. Castration can reduce some excitement and behavioural issues which are encountered with male dogs. When a female dog gets spayed, the vet takes out her reproductive organs (the uterus and the ovaries). The ovaries produce oestrogen, and are now no longer part of her body, hence major drops in the hormones and related triggers. Please be aware that these findings are based on my own research.

Is there a Diagnosis test which can confirm CECS?

The diagnosis of CECS is currently one of exclusion of other causes so the vet may wish to run blood and urine tests, carry out a full neurological examination and possibly do further tests to check for causes of epilepsy including electric recordings of the brain or MRI scans. A range of tests such as x-rays, endoscopy etc. may be needed to assess for intestinal and back disease. The condition is easily confused with epilepsy, back problems and even gut problems such as irritable bowel disease. It has been reported that a raised level of enzymes has been found when a liver function test has been performed but this has not been found in all cases.

Would Gaviscon, Buscopan or other digestion products help when the trigger is diet related?

My own research has found that in some cases of CECS that some digestion aid products have helped where diet has been the trigger or when your dog is experiencing a grumbly tummy. Prebiotics alongside probiotics can be beneficial too.

What is the difference between Buscopan and Gaviscon?

Gaviscon stops acid reflux by forming a film on top of the stomach's acids, preventing it from rising up the gullet. Buscopan isn't an antacid. It's a muscle relaxant/ antispasmodic to ease bowel spasms. It's taken reactively when symptoms are present rather than as a preventive measure.

Does Manuka honey help?

As with most supplements Manuka honey contains a lot of health benefits which are seen in humans and animals. Honey benefits dogs in numerous ways. Topically it heals wounds. Internally, it provides numerous sources of nutrients, such as vitamins A, B complex, C, D, E and K, plus minerals such as calcium, magnesium, and more. It helps dogs with allergies, fights infections, and helps with digestive problems.

Due to its antibacterial properties, honey benefits dogs who are suffering from gastroenteritis problems caused by overgrowth of harmful bacteria, such as gastritis, Inflammatory Bowel Disease (IBD), colitis, and so on.

Researchers are aware that when a CECS dog is having an episode that using honey on their gums can elevate the length of an episode. Again, this does not work for every CECS sufferer.

Manuka, as with all honey, contains a high sugar content so it could be that your dog's sugar levels do drop before the onset of an episode. Please be aware if your dog suffers from diabetes or is overweight, it's best to consult your veterinarian before giving Manuka to your dog. Manuka is not recommended for dogs under a year of age. Manuka may contain bacteria that your puppy isn't ready to fight off.

Unfortunately, we do not know and it would be very hard to monitor what changes in your dog's chemistry is taking place before a full-blown episode. What we do know is that tests carried out afterwards usually come back as normal or with a slightly raised liver reading.

Prescribed medication

Do prescribed epilepsy medications help CECS sufferers?

In some cases, prescribed medication from the vet do work to control episodes in dogs. This is not the case with all CECS sufferers. You also have to take into account whether the side effects from the medication could have an impact on your dog's health as well as their mental awareness. Common treatments prescribed:

- †Diazepam -Its known by the brand name Valium, is a drug that can be used in dogs as an anti-anxiety medication, a muscle relaxant, a treatment for seizures, and medicine for other conditions. It works by promoting gamma-aminobutyric acid (GABA) in the dog's brain, which blocks neurotransmitters that cause excitement.

- Phenobarbitone (sometimes abbreviated as Pb or Phb) is one of the medications most commonly used to treat seizures in dogs because it is relatively inexpensive, easy to **use** and effective in 60 to 80% of dogs with idiopathic epilepsy. In addition to being used on a daily basis to prevent seizures, Phenobarbital can be used to stop seizures in progress. Phenobarbital's peak activity occurs 4-8 hours after the pill is given. *While Pb is not FDA approved (USA) for use in dogs, it is one of two first choices for veterinarians and its use is accepted practice. Phenobarbital comes in liquid or tablet form and is available both from a veterinarian and from a regular pharmacy by prescription. When Phenobarbital is started, it takes 1 to 2 weeks to reach a stable blood level. Until that period has passed, it cannot be fully relied upon to prevent seizures.

- Valproic Acid - This medication is effective in humans with all types of seizures; however, it is metabolized very quickly in dogs and therefore its use is limited. Valproic Acid is primarily used in combination with other drugs such as Phenobarbital. Potential side effects include loss of hair and liver disease.

- Potassium bromide, sometimes abbreviated as KBr, is one of the traditional anticonvulsant medications used to treat canine and feline epilepsy. It is frequently used together with Phenobarbital but may be used by itself to control seizure activity as well. When starting potassium bromide, your vet might recommend an initial dose that is higher than the recommended maintenance dose. This is called a "loading dose" and it may be given over a one to five-day period. Once your pet is started on potassium bromide, you should not suddenly stop giving the medication unless advised by your veterinarian. If potassium bromide can or should be discontinued, it is best to slowly taper the dosage. Blood tests should be monitored periodically while your pet is receiving potassium bromide. Levels of bromide in the blood can be measured and may be recommended. Other blood testing, including liver enzymes and potassium levels, may be recommended as well.

- Levetiracetam - The most common side effects associated with this drug are drowsiness and loss of appetite, which are most commonly experienced in cats. Levetiracetam is commonly used in tandem with other anti-seizure medications because it allows the dosage of the other drugs to be decreased.

- Pexion – It's a treatment for dogs with primary epilepsy. It acts on a specific receptor in the brain cells to reduce the amount of excessive electrical activity present. In this way, like all epilepsy treatments, Pexion acts to reduce the number of seizures that your dog has and their impact on your dog's life.

  †The use of diazepam per rectum (RDZ) in the home to control generalized cluster seizures in 11 dogs diagnosed with idiopathic epilepsy was evaluated over a 16-month period. All dogs had a prior history of clusters of generalized seizures and were treated with multiple antiepileptic drugs. Owners were instructed to administer diazepam injectable solution (5 mg/mL) per rectum to their dogs at a dose of 0.5 mg/kg when an initial generalized seizure occurred and when a second or third generalized seizure occurred within 24 hours of the first seizure. Seizure activity was recorded by owners in a daily log before the onset of RDZ use and for the duration of RDZ use, which ranged from 57 to 464 days (median = 157 days). The median age at which the first seizure occurred and the median age at the time of enrollment in the study were 19 and 42 months, respectively. All 11 dogs were treated with phenobarbital, with 10 dogs receiving concomitant bromide therapy. No significant correlation between the duration of the first, second, or third antiepileptic drug therapy and the change in the number of cluster seizure events before or after use of RDZ was found. Comparisons of seizure activity were done for the same time interval before and after the onset of RDZ availability. A significant decrease in the total number of seizure events and the total number of cluster seizures events was found after RDZ availability. Similarly, a significant difference in the average number of seizures per cluster seizure event and the total number of isolated seizure events occurred before and after RDZ therapy

  † Podell M Ohio State University, Department of Veterinary Clinical Sciences, College of Veterinary Medicine, Columbus 43210, USA

Does Dr Bach's rescue remedy help?

Dogs have emotions too, just like humans. The only difference is that dogs cannot tell us how they are feeling. We then have to rely on identifying the changes are dogs maybe going through.

Most but not all border terriers that suffer from CECS show signs of fear, stress, excitement and to any change around them and can be very clingy to their owners.

Usually before an episode the dog sometimes displays similar behaviour patterns. These can be

- Excessive licking of paws

- Stretching or dragging themselves along the floor

- Trembling

- Loud intestinal noises

- Not being able to settle

When a dog begins an episode, some can become shocked and start to panic. They lose control of their muscles and they start to cramp up. A dog can show their anxieties which can be very distressing for its owner.

A flower remedy can be very useful before, during and after an episode. Owners usually try the Dr Bach's rescue remedy. Not all dogs respond to the rescue remedy.

To help restore the mental imbalance I looked at each of the Bach remedies, and then made a recipe up which covers most of the symptoms and triggers suffered by CECS dogs. The remedy is very effective for dogs suffering from a variety of problems and can be used as a general anti stress or calming tonic in all kinds of situations. The remedy can be rubbed into the gums or applied to the skin. Research has shown that the use of the CECS flower remedy can alleviate some of the triggers and symptoms.

Does golden paste work?

Turmeric powder is a bright yellow powder made by dry grinding of mature turmeric rhizomes (underground stems). The use of turmeric for colouring and flavouring food, for cosmetic purposes and for medicinal properties dates back to the ancient Vedic culture of India.

Golden paste has been used for dogs who suffer from CECS. Not much research has been done to know whether it has any benefits to the condition whether it reduces the number of episodes a dog may have.

The benefits of using Turmeric are:

- It's a natural detox

- It can be used as an anti-inflammatory and an antibacterial

- It can help aid heart disease and maintain liver health

- It can reduce blood clots that can lead to strokes and heart attacks by thinning the blood

- It can offer allergy relief

- Has been used in the treatment of epilepsy

- Natural pain relief

The downside to using Turmeric:

- Stomach upset, dizziness and nausea to start

- worsening gallbladder problems

- increased occurrence of bruising

- decreased blood sugar

- iron deficiency

- A smell similar to cat pee has been reported when using on your dog

- The dosage needs to be correct for the weight of your dog otherwise you could cause digestion and bowel problems.

Is coconut oil beneficial when managing CECS?

The latest trend in dog health care is adding coconut oil to their diet. Though it has been seen beneficial in humans, including everything from weight loss to a boosted immune system. It is considered anti-inflammatory, antiviral and antifungal. Some studies show that topical use of coconut oil may help against bacteria and viruses in humans with atopic dermatitis.

Coconut oil can be used as a treatment but like most supplements and treatments caution should be used due to the overall fat in the diet and it may not be suitable for some dogs.

Coconut oil should not be used if your dog suffers from pancreatitis or hyperlipidaemia (elevated levels of lipids or fats in the blood). Oral use can be very controversial between the holistic approach and conventical medicine. Topical use of coconut oil may benefit dry, itchy, irritated skin as well as crusty noses and pads

Coconut oil is also believed to beneficial for pets with inflammatory bowel disease and cognitive dysfunction. Caution should be used, however, for the same reasons stated above.

Topical use of coconut oil may benefit dry, itchy, irritated skin as well as crusty noses and pads.

We may eventually find it helpful in pets with other medical conditions, but there are just not enough studies to prove that yet and the risks may outweigh the benefit for many individuals.

You will find that the internet could be misleading with claims that Coconut oil can cure or reduce:

- Cancer prevention

- Dental calculus and periodontal disease prevention

- Weight loss

- Thyroid dysfunction

- Dry skin

- Wound healing

- Atopic dermatitis

- Inflammatory bowel disease

- Lymphangiectasis (poor bowel absorption)

- Cognitive dysfunction

While conducting my research into CECS I have found that the oral use of coconut oil could exacerbate the digestive issues encountered with some CECS sufferers.

Dental Hygiene

Is dental hygiene a factor when considering CECS?

Yes, I believe that if your dog's teeth and mouth are healthy that there is less chance of your dog digesting toxins and bacteria.

A dog with periodontal disease is prone to develop bacterial infection. Bacteria from a tooth abscess, for example, can easily gain access into the blood stream. If the number of bacteria is high, or if a dog has a compromised immune system, the bacterial infection can easily affect important body organs, such as:

- The Heart

Bacteria in the blood stream can gain access to the heart, causing a serious bacterial infection to the heart valve - a condition known as Bacterial Endocarditis (an infection of the heart valves) which can be fatal. In addition, some bacteria found in a dog's mouth are "sticky" and tend to adhere to the artery walls. If regular dental care is not given to a dog, therefore, this type of bacteria can accumulate along the artery walls, making them thicker and narrower for blood to pass through. As a result, heart disease can occur.

- The Kidneys

The kidneys filter out waste products and toxins from the blood to the urine. They also trap circulating bacteria. If the number of bacteria in the blood is high, bacterial infection can easily occur in the kidneys causing kidney damage. It is not uncommon that a dog with kidney problem recovers after proper dental treatment has been carried out.

- The Liver and Pancreas

Bacteria from canine dental problems can also affect the liver, causing hepatitis, and the pancreas, causing pancreatitis.

- Other Organs

Every other tissue and organ that has a blood supply (e.g. the lungs, the brain, muscles, etc.) is potentially at risk from bacterial infection spread by blood.

- Inhaled Infection

Canine dental problems can also cause inhaled infection. As a dog with periodontal disease inhales, bacteria can be carried down the airways. In a healthy dog or if the number of bacteria is small, the dog's defence mechanism may fend off any bacterial infection. However, if the immune system is compromised, or if the dog is already suffering from some form of respiratory disease such as bronchitis, or if the number of bacteria is high, then bacterial infection may take hold, wreaking havoc on the respiratory system.

- Ingestion of Toxins

Finally, if a dog has periodontal disease, over time the bacteria in his saliva will produce toxins. These toxins can easily be ingested by the dog when he swallows. When the toxins reach the stomach, not all of them can be destroyed by gastric acid. As a result, stomach problems such as gastritis may occur. It is therefore a rather common phenomenon for dogs with periodontal disease to have upset tummy.

Common conditions found in dogs.

- Gingivitis - inflammation of the gums.

- Periodontitis - a general term for a disease of the oral cavity that attacks the gum and bone and delicate tissues around the teeth.
- Pyorrhoea - inflammation of the gums and tooth sockets, often leading to loosening of the teeth and accompanied by pus.
- Plaque - the first build-up of material adhering to tooth enamel. Composed of a mix of intercellular matrix of bacteria, salivary polymers, remnants of epithelial cells and white blood cells, it can cause caries, calculi build-up and periodontal disease.
- Calculus (Tartar) - calcium carbonate and calcium phosphate combined with organic material, deposited on the surface of the tooth.

Drinking water

Can drinking water affect a dog with CECS?

I believe that water quality, where you live and the temperature of water can have an impact on a dog who suffers with CECS.

The practice of making water safe to drink actually involves adding large amounts of extremely poisonous chemicals to it. Key scientists are now providing evidence that long-term ingestion of small amounts of chemicals like these could be the cause of some major health problems in humans as well as our pets.

Here is a list of just a few of the chemicals routinely added to our water supply:

- Liquified chlorine
- Fluor silicic acid
- Aluminium sulphate
- Calcium hydroxide
- Sodium silico fluoride

Contaminants in Tap Water

Tap water is treated with a large number of chemicals in order to kill bacteria and other microorganisms. In addition, it may contain other undesirable contaminants like toxic metal salts, hormones and pesticides, or it may become contaminated by chemicals or microbes within pipes (e.g. lead, bacteria, protozoa).

Would it be better to used filtered water?

Water filters remove chlorine and some pesticides. However, they do not remove fluoride, hormones, toxic metal salts and other chemicals.

Recently a study has shown that distilled water removes all impurities from the water including salts which can be harmful and can cause unrelated epilepsy seizures, arthritis and joint related problems.

Mineral salts cannot be processed correctly by the kidneys so the salts may be trapped in tissues and deposited in the joints, kidneys and liver. All dogs who suffer from Arthritis should have distilled water to improve their health, it will dissolve all salt deposits within 3-4 weeks. Most owners notice a big improvement in their pet's health within 6-8 weeks and your pet will suffer with less pain. They are expensive but worth every penny in my opinion. It would be another way to make sure your dog was not consuming toxins or salts which could be contributing to a CECS episode.

Can CECS kill my dog?

There is no evidence to date that a dog has died from a CECS episode or any symptoms related to CECS.

How do I know what the 'Triggers' are?

Unfortunately, it is a case of monitoring your dog's diet, environment and general health to find the cause of the triggers. Not all dogs are the same and each one may have a different trigger.

Can my other dog catch CECS?

No, it would be classed as a disease rather than a syndrome. The difference being that a syndrome is a set of medical signs and symptoms that are correlated with each other and, often, with a particular disorder. A "disease" has a pathological cause such as bacteria or a virus.

What if my dog isn't gluten sensitive?

My research has shown that not all CECS cases have an intolerance to Gluten. It has also shown that the Natural restore supplement can help some dogs overcome gluten intolerance.

My dog doesn't have digestive issues?

Not all dogs show the same symptoms. Some suffer noisy tummies while others do not. Most dogs digest their food at different rates and this could be due to exercise, environment and the diet they are on.

What food and things should I avoid to help my dog and what could I give to help elevate the symptoms?

A diet must be tailormade for that individual dog. You need to take into consideration when choosing a diet

- They don't have any allergies or intolerances.

- You must meet the needs of your dog (whether they are working terriers, show or pets)

- How much exercise your dog gets (to meet their energy needs).

- The correct amount for the weight of your dog

- A good healthy diet which is palatable for your dog rather than it being more convenient for the owner

How early does this start, and how old is the latest age he/she can be triggered CECS can develop at any age?

It has been reported dogs as young as 6 months have been affected but the usual age is 2-3 years in most cases. If you have an elderly dog who is presenting similar symptoms to CECS you must seek veterinary advice as soon as possible due to other illnesses and diseases which are encountered with the more senior dog.

Is there any medication from my vet for this?

Due to the lack of knowledge and not knowing the true cause or triggers there is no known prescribed treatment for CECS. Your vet may advise administrating a Rectal Diazepam or when your dog is actually having a full-blown episode. It helps relax the muscles and can shorten the length of the cramps. I advise that this treatment should only be used in more server episodes which are lasting over 10 minutes.

Can rawhide chews be a trigger for a CECS episode?

Rawhide is not a by-product of the beef industry and it is not made of dehydrated meat. It is actually a by-product of the leather industry.

Usually the cattle hide is shipped from the slaughter house to tanneries for processing. These hides are treated with a chemical to help preserve the product in transport. The hides are them soaked and treated with either ash-lye solution or a highly toxic recipe of sodium sulphide liming. This helps to remove hair and fats from the hides. They are then treated with a chemical that will help puff the hide making it easier to split into thin layers. The outer layer is used in the clothing and furniture industry and the inner layer is used for rawhides. The inner hide is then washed and whitened using a solution of hydrogen peroxide or bleach which will remove the smell of rotting putrid leather. These white sheets are then basted, smoked and tinted using dyes and flavours. To make them appear white they are coated with titanium oxide. They are then pressed into different shapes which may appeal to the owner. A study was conducted by into the process of rawhide and they found traces of Arsenic, Lead, Mercury, Chromium salts, Formaldehyde and other toxic chemicals. An investigation by the Humane Society International stated in a report that some rawhide chews are in fact skin from slaughtered dogs in Thailand and China.

Rawhide chews start out hard but as your dog chews them they become softer and eventually turn into a slimy piece of gum. At this point they become useless as a dental chew and do not benefit your dog. They in fact become a chocking and intestinal obstruction hazard. Once in the gut the digestion process can be put under strain to try to digest the rawhide. The liver and kidneys can become compromised due to the chemical toxins.

The bile duct starts producing too much bile which may cause cramping of the stomach and vomiting.

Can my dog have several different triggers that cause his episodes?

Each dog is different and they may have one to several triggers. It is a process of elimination. By keeping a daily diary of weather conditions, general health, diet, environmental issues and other causes which may trigger a CECS symptoms or episode can be very helpful for you to determine what may be causing the problem.

Are Border Terriers the only breed that gets this?

My research has shown that CECS mainly affects the Border Terrier but it has been reported that other breeds are suffering similar symptoms to the condition. I have come across Border Collie's, pugs, poodles and Labradors which have presented CECS.

Should I be concerned over anaesthetic?

My research has shown that no complications or episodes have been reported while dogs are under anaesthetic. My own dog Josh has had 3 operations where I have been present and all monitored readings were normal through-out the procedure. Afterwards, he did seem to take a little longer to come around from the anaesthetic but did not have an episode and showed signs of being ill afterwards.

Can vaccinations and boosters trigger CECS episode?

There is quite a lot of controversy surrounding vaccinations and boosters over the recent years. This is due to having the technologies in science of today and knowing the affects they are having on our dogs.

Recent studies have found that boosters are increasingly associated with chronic disorders such as reoccurring skin and anal gland problems as well as seizures in some dogs.

In the UK owners are asked to vaccinate their dogs from 8 weeks of age. They have one initial vaccination which is a broad-side of a powerful multiple vaccines and then another between 2 to 4 weeks after. They then request that the dog has a booster each year. If you want to board your dogs at a kennels or take your dog abroad you are required to have annual boosters.

In recent years a steady stream of evidence from leading researchers have challenged the effeteness and scientific validity of the practice. Experts say that almost without exceptions there is no need for the annual boosters.

Immunity to viruses last for years or for the life of a dog, and most vaccinations to most bacterial pathogens produces long term protection.

The role that vaccines play is preventing, controlling and eliminating diseases. This practice would be more effective if more unvaccinated pets were vaccinated and less concentration on already vaccinated pets. A simple test can be conducted on your dog to determine which individual vaccine they may require if any. Researchers have concluded that the annual boosters should in fact be given once every three years (if required) and that older dogs should not need them. They do advise to monitor antibody levels annually as a precaution.

My own research has found that boosters, kennel cough vaccine, worming products and flea treatments as a trigger to CECS episodes. Episodes usually happen within 2-6 weeks after any of those treatments.

A reason for this could be due to an accumulation of chemicals and toxins which could disrupt the normal function of the digestive and immune system. This could in turn affect the kidney and liver functions and toxins could seep into the blood and contaminate the brain causing nerve problems.

Are worming and flea treatments safe for my CECS dog?

My research has found that some products do affect CECS dogs but not all. The less chemicals and toxins we expose our dogs to the better it is for them. The key to managing CECS is to remove all toxins whether manmade or through the digestion process.

Preventing fleas and ticks is an important part of caring for your pet and keeping yourself (and home) pest-free.

"In addition to being a nuisance, (fleas and ticks) can transmit parasites and numerous disease-carrying organisms, with illnesses which could range from mild to life-threatening

Left untreated, fleas can cause skin rashes, anaemia and bacterial diseases while ticks can be a carrier of Lyme disease, a dangerous and potentially damaging condition for your pet, and for humans too. Fleas can be picked up from the outdoors, other pets and indoor areas where fleas may be present. They reproduce rapidly and can be a major problem for people's clothing, furniture, and hair in addition to their pet. Ticks are generally picked up outdoors, especially in heavily wooded areas.

There are so many products on the market at the moment that it can be like a minefield out there as to which one you need to choose for your pet. It is alleged that some scientists have gone on to say that the flea, the tick and the common worm have adapted quite well to the chemical products we use for our dogs and the product may not be strong enough to prevent our dogs from catching parasites. Most products on the market are chemical based and sometimes the dosage suggested may harm your dog or not even protect it due to the wrong amount given to your pet. Most manufacturers use a suggested dosage which goes on weight. This can be very varied and can be very confusing for owners. The weight range is usually 2kg to 10kg, 10 kg to 20kg, 20kg to 40 kg and the 40kg to 60kg. Personally, the range is too varied. Surely a small dog at 2 kg should not be having the same dosage of chemicals as a 10kg dog.

So which product to go for?

Most flea & tick treatments require applying the medication between your pet's shoulder blades, or at the base of their neck. They are absorbed by the animal's oil and sweat glands in the skin and help your pet repel fleas and ticks within 24 hours. Nearly all flea and tick treatments are chemical based and can cause hair loss, irritation and in some cases vomiting, cramping and being off colour.

Tablets from the vet dissolve in the gut and purge a high shot of chemicals which is distributed through the digestive system. This can cause colitis and irritation of the pancreas and upper bowel. The one where you put drops at the back of the neck again is highly concentrated and works by soaking into the fat cells and then it's distributed throughout the major organs and fed into the blood system. This too can cause skin allergies, fur loss, digestion problems and cramping.

Most shop bought flea and worming products do not contain Fipronil. It is a proven fact that this chemical needs to be in the certain treatments for it to work correctly. Fipronil is widely used at the moment but research so far has shown that the common parasite is building up a resistant to it.

Natural or chemical based collars are quite popular due to the cost. In my opinion they very seldom work, they have a very short shelf life and when the product is used it is only targeting one area which is around the neck. If your dog decides to remove the collar and eat it you will have to seek medical help otherwise your dog maybe at risk of poisoning.

The one I usually suggest is an all-natural ingredient which can be added to their food in small doses and it is absorbed by digestion process and then distributed through the kidneys, pancreas and liver via the blood. This in turn makes the rich blood taste repulsive to the parasite. They usually leave the host and try to find a better candidate to feed on.

The natural wormer works by gently rubbing the bowel lining to stop worms from attaching to it. These products are naturally based and it is very rare that it causes allergies of other problems which are encountered by chemical-based ones.

How do I go about getting a diagnosis if my vets don't find anything wrong?

Once your vet rules out other illnesses and diseases he may then look at the breed individually for other causes of your dog's condition.

Is there a difference between CECS and paroxysmal gluten-sensitive dyskinesia(PGSD)?

My research has shown a similarity between both conditions and I feel that some dogs are being misdiagnosed as having CECS when they are actually intolerant to Gluten. I have been treating dogs who can tolerate gluten but still have the symptoms of CECS.

Has there been any evidence that anal gland issues are linked to CECS?

I'm not sure whether there is a link but my own findings on the subject it does appear that in some cases but not all that anal glands can be over producing and then compacting when CECS is present. Anal glands are openings on each side of a canine's anus, beneath the skin and leading to the sac openings are tiny tubes that release a pungent smelling brown liquid substance whenever the dog defecates. The anal sacs then are considered scent glands that are primarily used to release that strong smell unique to each dog and needed to mark a territory.

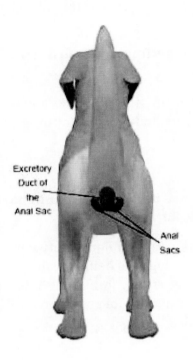

Excretory
Duct of
the
Anal Sac

Anal
Sacs

They also help the dog's body regulate hard stools and eliminate toxins. In other words, these sacs are quite an important part of your pet's digestive and elimination function.

What happens is that when a stool is passed, this puts a bit of pressure on the sacs and triggers the release of the noxious smell. That scent is then used by dogs as a way to communicate with each other and, as mentioned above, mark a territory. This is also the reason why canines sniff each other's butts. They are simply trying to learn which smell belongs to which dog. Any irregularities must be treated right away before the condition worsens.

There are several ways you can tell if there is a problem with the anal glands. These can be

- Scooting – your dog dragging his rectal area along the floor (this may be a sign of worms or other infections too, so it is best to confirm)

- Constant biting or licking of his anus or the base of his tail

- Bad smell is coming off from his rear end (might be accompanied by pus-looking discharge)

- Obvious constipation when defecating

- Other behaviour that shows your dog is experiencing discomfort in the anal region

Some owners describe a pungent smell when their dog is experiencing a CECS episode. This could be due to the cramping muscles which may express the glands.

Since the anal glands are an important part of a dog's body detoxification, if liver toxicity is high, the sacs will often become inflamed and then problems arise.

- colitis (bacteria seeping back into the bowels and contaminating the colon).
- Injury due to rubbing the affected area on a rough service.
- Compacted anal glands will cause pain and discomfort.
- Toxins are not being removed from the body

Regular checks on the anal glands is very important for heathy dogs as well as CECS dogs.

Why don't more vets know of this condition?

Some vets are aware of CECS but unfortunately some vets are misdiagnosing the condition as epilepsy.

Is there a cure for CECS?

At the present there is no cure for CECS but there is a way of managing the illness and by way of diet and removing possible triggers.

Where can I find help and support from other owners whose dogs have this? Jan Gale and a friend set up a Facebook group so that owners to share their experience of living with a CECS dog. The group has been a valuable source of information and has over 2000 members. For more information visit https://www.facebook.com/groups/2877304097/

Is CECS hereditary?

Research has shown that in some cases that if one of the parents show signs of CECS that there is a chance that any siblings may also present the symptoms.

Will my dog grow out of CECS?

This is a condition which can change at any time. Some dogs may only have one full blown episode in their lifetime while others may have 2-3 each month. With good management through diet and reducing the triggers your dog could have less episodes.

What is the best diet for this condition?

Due to each dog having their own requirements and needs what diet may be good for one dog may not be good for another. Gluten free does seem to help some dogs who suffer from this condition but not all.

What do I do if my dog is having an episode?

All dogs respond differently when having an episode. I would recommend you leave your dog where it is rather than trying to move them unless any harm can come to them. Moving a dog who has cramp could cause them to feel more uncomfortable. Just sit beside them and place your hand on them and try to reassure them with your voice that the episode will pass soon. Try to maintain eye contact with them and gentle rub their head and tummy. Try to slow your breathing down and relax. Hopefully your dog will feel this and feel more at ease.

Will it affect the general health and wellbeing of my dog?

There is no evidence that a dog who has CECS cannot live a long and otherwise a healthy life. Some dogs who suffer from CECS do have bouts of colitis and other symptoms associated with the condition. These can be easily managed through diet and prebiotics.

Will my dog have these episodes often?

Each dog is different and there is no limit to how many episodes your dog will have in their lifetime. If your dog's trigger is heat you may find it harder to manage the condition due to environmental factors. Excitement, stress, illness may also be a trigger and once again it is unlikely to predict if and when an episode will occur.

Why do a lot of vets think it is epilepsy?

This is because CECS has the characteristics and resembles epilepsy but your dog is conscious through-out the episode. Today more vets are being made aware of Canine Epileptoid Cramping Syndrome. With this knowledge and better understanding they can offer advice for those who suffer with this condition.

What is SLEM?

† Spongiform Leukoencephalomyelopathy (SLEM) is a hereditary disease of Border Terriers. When the pups begin to stand and attempt to walk, they show an uncontrollable shaking of their hind limbs causing a characteristic "rump shaking". As the pups develop, the shaking affects the entire body and their coordination is poor. Most pups are euthanized due to a poor quality of life but there are reports of dogs improving with intensive nursing care.

The nerve cells in the brain communicate with each other through electrical signals. These signals are conveyed from one area of the brain to another through extensions of the cell called axons. Like an electrical cord, the axons must be insulated to keep the electrical signals from shorting out. The insulation of the axons is called myelin. If the brain is cut at a post-mortem exam, the myelin gives the bundles of axons running from one area of the brain to another a glistening, white colour, so these areas are called "white matter". If the insulating myelin does not form properly, then areas of the brain cannot communicate with each other efficiently. The poor communication affects the ability of the puppy to control movements resulting in the signs of SLEM.

When post-mortem examinations were performed on affected pups, they found that the myelin had not formed properly in areas of the brain and spinal cord. In a normal pup, the dense insulation appears purplish-pink when the tissues are stained for examination under the microscope. In the affected pups, there are basically holes where the insulation should be giving the tissue a spongy look. So, the condition is termed spongiform leukoencepahomyelopathy: spongiform (like a sponge) leuko (white)- encephalo (brain)- myelo (spinal cord)- pathy (disease). We call it by the initials SLEM.

† Information taken from University of Missouri,

Is CECS directly linked to a celiac type disorder?

While dogs in general don't suffer from true celiac disease (with the possible exception of Red Setters), gluten can be a problematic ingredient for many dogs, and can cause problems like gastro-intestinal upset similar to that seen in humans, as well as itchy skin and ear infections. My research has shown that most dogs who suffer from CECS are fit and healthy between episodes and rarely show signs of other illnesses.

Why does my dog have them on waking up?

We are unable to monitor our dogs before an episode (blood tests and other diagnostic tests) we cannot tell what changes your dog's body is going through. May be a dog's sugar levels may drop while resting and on waking up the body goes into a mini shock syndrome. What we do know is that administrating honey, flower remedies and pressing on a pressure point GV26 is the most important one, as it can help stop a seizure. It is where the nose meets the upper lip (immediately below the nostrils).

Can a dog have CECS if it has purely intestinal issues and no neurological signs?

Some dogs may experience some of the symptoms associated with CECS but these problems must be addressed by your vet. There could be other issue's which may be going off like intolerance to gluten, foods, allergies, pancreatitis, colitis and other digestive conditions.

Can stress, either physical (illness, emergency surgery or elective surgery) or emotional (anxiety or excitement) trigger the episodes?

Yes, my research has shown that these conditions can be a trigger. Keeping a diary can be helpful to pin point certain situations which you may want to avoid. Try Flower remedies and other natural products to help your dog relax when faced with these situations.

Can heat be a trigger, and if so why?

My research has shown that heat and cold can be a trigger for a full-blown episode. Environmental changes either hot and cold weather and indoor heating may affect the digestion process. For digestion to take place and run smoothly the body must create the right environment for the breakdown of food as well as extracting nutrients. If there are any changes through heat or cold I believe the digestion process could be slowed down so accumulation of gases may be more present when digesting (causing a bloat affect, gases could be absorbed into the blood stream and then the brain). The digestion process could be speeded up to the extent that food is not correctly digested so it causes a colitis affect.

Is there any lasting damage caused?

My research has shown that a dog may return to normal after an episode. Some owners have reported their dog being tired and the need to pass urine or empty their bowels. No lasting damage neurological or physically has been found to date.

Can travelling in the car trigger an episode?

Yes, it can. Travel sickness seems to be more common than what it was a few years back. Whether it's due to the technology cars are using nowadays I'm not sure. Some CECS dogs can find travelling quite stressful which can bring on an episode. Travel sickness is all to do with the inner ear and balance. Dogs are the same as humans, we both process sight, balance, and motion. Most dogs when travelling in a car cannot see the outside of the car and if they can it is a blur. This sends mixed messages to the brain which triggers a process of movement and balance. Unless the eyes can focus on the horizon it cannot process what is happening. It's this which causes the car sickness. You would of all seen dogs hanging out of car windows. They are not getting a free blow-dry but they are fixing their eyes on the horizon. I suggest you buy a booster seat for your dog so it can see out of the front window or side windows. Keep the window down by a couple of inches. Some dogs prefer to be in the back so they can see out of the back window. (Less movement for the brain to process). You could also try a relaxer or calmer but this isn't a quick fix or a one off. Two days before you travel your dog needs to be prepared. Start any treatment a couple of days before you travel for the dog to feel the full benefit.

Could depression be a trigger for CECS?

Dogs like humans fall ill to any number of diseases. The health issues may be social, physical or emotional. One recent concern is dog depression. Dogs can suffer from this emotional ailment. Talk to your vet and a behavioural psychologist to see if your dog is depressed. If this proves true, take the appropriate steps to help him or her return to the vitality that should be their life.

There is little doubt that dogs can and do suffer from the same emotional problems befalling human beings. Dogs of all types and ages can exhibit characteristics of several of the more common problems. These include anxiety, obsessive, compulsive order and phobias. They may begin licking their paws for no apparent reason.

Dog depression is, at its simplest, an expression of sadness. The dog is not content or happy. He or she is nervous, anxious and obviously depressed. Your dog may also lose their appetite for food.

A depressed dog may sleep more and seem lethargic. Your dog may seem down and not excited by life as they would have yesterday, last week or last month. If this change in behaviour often takes place without any sign of a physical problem or health issue, it may be depression.

Some common causes:

- Moving home
- deceased family member
- deceased pet
- Changing your dog's routine
- Trauma including accidents
- Changes in your dog's diet
- New feeding and water bowls
- Changes in where your dog sleeps
- A new partner or changes in your sexual behaviour
- Taking a different route while out walking
- Adding another family member
- Yours and family members moods and behaviour

The biggest and most common cause is usually down to your moods and your behaviour. In some instances, the advice may be directed to you. Dogs are empathic. They feel what you feel. The closer they are to a person, the more likely he or she will react to your own moods. If your dog is depressed because you are depressed, see and talk to your own doctor.

The good news is unlike humans, dogs live more for the moment. Although depression can linger for weeks or even months in dogs, the feelings and related symptoms are usually temporary. Most dogs will overcome the problems on their own. It may just take a bit of time for them to cope and adjust.

Diet

How can I tell if my dog is on the correct diet?

The appearance of your dog can tell you whether they are on the correct diet. The skin is the largest organ in the body and usually if there is a problem you tend to find the dog has dry, flaky or inflamed skin. The fur should be shiny and not dull in colour. The skin should be free from flea's, mites, ringworm and inflammatory allergies. The dog should appear happy, active and responsive. If your dog is showing signs of being irritable, dull appearing, hyperactive, nervous or restless it could be they are on the incorrect diet. If you change foods you should monitor our dog for several weeks afterwards to make sure they stay fit, healthy and happy.

If your dog is on the correct diet a properly functioning digestive system produces small amounts, well formed, dark in colour firm stools. The small amount tells you that the body's digestive system is extracting the right amount of nutrients, vitamins and minerals. The colour may indicate any food dyes, bleeding or at which the rate the food is being digested.

If the stools are soft the body may not be absorbing enough water from the diet. If this does happen your dog is at risk of dehydration. If the stools are too firm they may cause constipation and your dog may be uncomfortable. That tells you that the dog is not getting enough water in their diet. Poor quality food can result in undigested food passing into the large intestine. If it does fermentation from bacteria can produce gases and make your dog feel uncomfortable and cause loud abdominal noises.

If the intestines are inflamed the stools will be abnormal and your dog may pass blood. If your dog has any issues with their liver or pancreas they can cause digestive imbalance and produce abnormal stools. Veterinary advice is needed in any situation where there is a change in bowel movements.

How do I get my dog to eat?

Dogs are really good at clearing their dishes when it comes to food – The day will come when your dog decides to stop eating. There can be a number of reasons why your dog decides to change its eating habits. Firstly, you have to rule out any medical reason why this has happened. Some reasons are a bad tooth or teeth, gum disease, thrush (candidiasis) or a digestive problem.

If your dog skips a couple of meals this is not a problem for them but it does pose a big problem for us as owners. Alarm bells ring and you start panicking, it's at that point you start presenting your dog with all kinds of foods and treats which if eaten could result in an upset stomach and diarrhoea.

What you have to realise is that your dog has had a tailored diet to suit their needs and environment. For instance, I feed my dogs on raw, it gives them the correct amount of nutrition and they enjoy their meals. If I decided to feed them dry pet food it would cause an imbalance within the body and could result in diarrhoea and sickness. The reason: the digested system would have to process the food an entirely different way than it has been used to.

When making any change to your dog's diet it should be done gradually over a period of time. If your dog has been used to wet food and you give then give them dry food, it would mean your dog would have to drink more water, more water means the kidneys would have to work harder. The pancreas would now have to process more fats and proteins. The stomach its self would produce more bile and digestive juices which could make your dog feel as though its stomach is full and the liver itself would produce more enzymes. The bowel and gut are where the good and the bad bacteria live. They can live in harmony for years but as soon as there is a change in your dog's diets all hell can break loose and this could result in diarrhoea. All these conditions just mentioned can cause your dog to be in pain and to appear off colour. If you had stomach pain and was feeling under the weather would you eat a Sunday dinner? I don't think many of you would. Most of us can have days where we don't eat properly and are quite happy at snacking on bits and pieces. Some dogs want to snack rather than eat a set meal. If that happens don't look at it as though it is a problem. If the dog walks away from its dish take it up until next feeding time. Your dog is not going to collapse and die of starvation if it hasn't eaten for a few days. If a dog is that hungry it would eat whatever you put in front of it.

We are to blame for a dog being a picky eater. Due to all the different products available on the market, we decide what we think is right for our dogs rather than choosing the correct diet for your dog. If we like gravy surely the dog would want gravy! We like crunchy food, they like crunchy foods! We prefer beef, they prefer beef. Many of us are programming our dogs to eat a diet which may not be suitable for their digestive systems.

If a dog stops eating there could be a physiological reason. If your dog was sick after eating a meal it can then associate food as a bad thing. We then realise the dog has stopped eating, what do we do? Make a grab for human food, we offer the dog tinned fish, fresh chicken, fresh beef, tinned soup, corned beef, sliced ham and you get the picture anything to tempt your dog to eat. We tend to forget that most of our foods are processed. The majority of it contains things which dogs are not use to digesting. They may contain salts, sugars and fats as well as vegetable proteins and other additives and preservatives. Again, this upsets the digestion process of the dog and usually causes other problems like dehydration due to the salts, high blood sugar readings and the liver and pancreas would be under a lot of pressure to process them.

In some of the above for mentioned foods, they contain a product called soy. Soy can be very harmful to dogs and can cause cramping of the stomach. If this happens usually an owner or a vet cannot physically see this happening. Blood test results show high enzymes which say's the liver is not functioning properly and the blood glucose level is high as well as some raise ketones in the urine.

So how do we overcome this problem? You have to go back to basics, treat your dog as though it was a puppy.

I suggest the first couple of meals be as bland as possible, i.e. Turkey, it has less fat than chicken, so it gives pancreas and the bile ducts a rest. Brown rice so that your dog feels full but in effect is light so it is less likely to be vomited back up. Some dogs do find it difficult to process rice so you can try Dried Smash potato. Smash contains a binding agent which is easy on the digestion and can help form firmer stools. A tablespoon of natural live yoghurt, this will help stabilise the good and bad bacteria making the stomach and the intestines more settled when food is present. You can also try white fish, keep away from oily fish. (You can also try baby food in jars, they are full of nutrients which are safe for your dog and will be gentle on the tummy). Give small meals at first, maybe 2 large tablespoons every 4 hours. If it eats in the kitchen try feeding your dog in another room. Try to relax and don't show your dog any concern if it doesn't eat. Try feeding your dog at the same time as yourself. It's better to eat as a pack than as an individual. Remember we are going back to puppy days when siblings ate together.

Food always tastes better to a dog if it's stolen. If your dog won't eat pretend to be preparing food and knock some turkey on the floor. Carry on doing what you're doing and ignore the dog. If the dog walks away from it leave it on the floor chances are the dog will be tempted back. Try putting their food on a plate; leave it somewhere so they can steal.

Once the dog's tummy has settled start to introduce the original food you gave them as a puppy. Add this slowly to the meals so that their digestive systems can adjust. Puppy food is ideal because it contains, vitamins and nutrients which are essential to maintaining the dog's health while they are off colour. After a few weeks introduce the adult food that your dog enjoyed and was healthy on. This process can take weeks or even months, don't make the mistake of trying to rush things otherwise you'll be back to square one.

It only takes one meal to upset your dog's digestive system but it can take over a month to correct it.

Only change your dog's diet if there is a medical reason to do so and then contact a canine nutritional advisor rather than a vet to help decide what diet your dog needs.

Understanding pet foods and choosing the right one for our dog.

It can be a mine field out there when it comes to choosing the right diet for your dog. We have dried food, tinned food, Raw and the dehydrated diet. We then have to decide whether to choose working dog, breed specific, special diet food, Gluten free, no gluten added, sterilised, low protein, high protein, sporting dog, no wheat, no grain, no added preservatives, no colourings and the list goes on.

Another choice we have to make is Brand and price according to our budget.

All dogs are different when it comes to feeding and you need to choose a diet which suits your dog. You have to take into consideration how much exercise they get, what allergies or intolerance they may have to ingredients and they age of the dog. Would you like your dog to be fed a chemical free diet, totally dry, semi moist, tinned or a natural diet.

- **Raw diet:** This diet if done correctly can be very beneficial to your dog. Some owners are put off by the idea of feeding raw meat due to harmful bacteria's. A dog's digestion is very different to ours and their digestion process is designed to eliminate these. Owners are frightened to feed their dogs bones in case they choke or will cause a blockage. You have to understand which types of bones are good and which bones you have to avoid. Try to keep away from weight bearing bones because these tend to be very strong and may damage your dog's teeth. Most raw pet food supplies offer raw mince which is easily digested by your dog. The majority of these minces do contain grinded bones as well as organs, meat, feathers, skin, intestines (containing content), fats as well as vegetables and fruit. Ground mince contains vital nutrients and vitamins which will cater for your dog's needs. Boned meat which can be chewed and digested easily are chicken and rabbit (these bones do not splinter if uncooked).

- **Soft moist food:** These foods are high in sugar, chemicals, colourings, propylene glycol and other additives to give them their shelf life and softness.

- **Dry combination "Generic Brands"** This food is usually cheap and contain fillers such as rice, potato and grains. They usually lack vital minerals which can result in a deficiency especially zinc. Some of these brands advertise that their products as 'No gluten added'. This means that they cannot guarantee that gluten has not been intentionally added.

- **Standard commercial diets:** These are an adequate diet for most, normal, healthy, young to middle aged dogs. They are not suitable for older dogs or dogs who are ill. They are made to be competitive and usually filled with preservatives and additives. Most contain colourings to make the owner think they look appealing for their dog.

- **Top shelf dried food:** These products contain quality ingredient but can still contain artificial preservatives and other chemical additives. Usually the kibble comes in a different size to cater for small to large breeds jaws.

- **Breed specific food:** The manufactures tailor makes a food for breeds who suffer from a specific trait. This range contains a multitude of formulas tailored to individual dog breeds. They use quality ingredient, protein sources, specific nutrients, and kibble designed with specific shape, size and texture for each dog breed's jaw structure and biting pattern.

- **Natural diet:** These products are usually made from the finest quality ingredients. They use vitamin C and Vitamin E as a natural preservative instead of using an artificial one. They have added minerals that contain a high level of amino acids so giving a better absorption rate. This is a good diet for all dogs, especially the elderly or ill dogs.

- **Homemade diet:** This is the best food you could feed your dog. The homemade diet is made from fresh meat, vegetables and other ingredient's. They are free from preservatives, colourings and fillers.

The sad truth is that it's impossible to say from the packaging alone whether some foods might contain artificial preservatives or not. This is because, while additives added by the manufacturers themselves have to be declared on the packaging, there is a legal loophole allowing artificial additives that were added to the ingredients before they reached the pet food factory to go undeclared. In fact, even if a food is littered with ingredients that have been individually treated with artificial preservatives before reaching the factory, the manufacturer can still legally claim that the food has 'no *added* preservatives' as they technically didn't add any.

Fresh meat (Beef, chicken, lamb, Rabbit)

These meats are high-quality ingredients which contain beneficial nutrients and should be the main ingredient in a dog's diet. Recently studies have shown an increase in some allergies towards these particular meats.

Duck, Turkey, Pork

These meats are easy to digest and are lower in fat than the above and they contain beneficial nutrients. Pork was once thought of as a problem for dogs. It is now wildly recognised by a nutritionist as a good palatable meat source. It can be very useful for allergy-prone dogs as it is impossible to be allergic to a food that they have not been exposed to. Uncooked pork is not advisable for a dog on a raw diet as it carries a higher risk of parasitic infection. Duck and Turkey are two of the easiest meats for a dog to digest. They are a good source of high-quality protein and contain vitamin A and vitamin B3 as well as a good source of several minerals. Turkey is lower in fat compared to chicken and is more palatable when dogs are ill.

Bone Meal/Fish meal

Both products are medium quality ingredients. They are both added to some dog's foods as a natural calcium and phosphorous supplements. The bone meal should be avoided if your dog has a particular allergy to certain meats. This is due to not knowing which kind of meat the meal comes from.

Liver

High-quality ingredient with some very beneficial nutrients. Nutrition varies from species to species but they are all good. They are rich in vitamin B12, vitamin A, copper, folate, riboflavin and selenium. It also contains zinc, vitamin C, B5 and B6, protein, niacin, phosphorous and iron. It is easily digestible and high palatable.

Meat Meal

This is another quality ingredient with beneficial nutrients. It is fine, dry brown powder which, for many years has been used to form the backbone of the dry food industry. It can be listed in a number of ways, with or without the animal source. Meat meal from the chicken would be labelled as chicken meal, dehydrated, or dried chicken. Meat meal is made from the parts of animals that are not consumed by humans. UK Food regulators say meat meal should be free from hair, bristles, feathers, horn, hoof, skin and the contents of the stomach and viscera. The general term 'meat meal' means that it could have come from any species of warm-blooded land animals. Broad terms like this are often used by dog food manufacturers instead of naming each ingredient either because the recipe changes between batches or the ingredients would put customers off. Another factor to take into consideration is that antioxidant must be added to the meat meal during its production in order to prevent it from becoming rancid. The most artificial antioxidant and commonly used in meat is the highly controversial and potentially harmful chemicals BHT, BHA and Propyl gallate. The main issue is that, since the antioxidants are added to the meat at the meat rendering plant long before it arrives at the dog food factory, the manufacturers do not need to declare them on the label. In fact, a food can contain any number of ingredients that have been pre-treated with artificial additives just as long as they don't add anymore themselves. For this reason, it's always important to look for foods that are guaranteed, free from Artificial antioxidants rather than Free from added artificial ingredients.

Tripe

Tripe is a high-quality ingredient and it contains beneficial nutrients. It can be used in its fresh form or as a pre-prepared dry meal. When it is listed on the labels as 'tripe' it usually refers to the fresh form. Tripe is the stomach of ruminating animals – usually cows and sheep. It is highly nutritional and is easily digestible. It is rich in protein, fat and is a good source of essential oils. Green tripe has not been cleaned, bleached or otherwise processed. Green tripe is unique because it contains high levels of probiotic including good bacteria and digestive enzymes that benefit the dog's digestion.

Crustaceans (shrimp, prawns, crabs etc)

Crustaceans are the most popular source of the joint supplement glucosamine, due to the very high concentration found in their shells. They are sometimes added directly to dog food and labelled as 'Crustaceans' or the glucosamine can be extracted through hydrolysis in which case it will appear as Glucosamine sulphate or Hydrolysed crustaceans.

Fish meal and fish derivatives

This is a low-grade source of ingredient and should be avoided. The EU defines 'Fish meal and fish derivatives fish or fish parts, fresh or preserved by appropriate treatments (chemicals added). The fish is usually very poor quality.

Fish oil

Fish oil should be part of your dog's diet due to the high levels of nutrients and vitamins. Fish oil comes from the processing of oily fish like tuna, sardines, salmon and mackerel. It provides energy, essential omega 3 and omega 6 oils. Fish oils are recommended for the prevention and treatment of joint problems, skin conditions, cardiovascular disease and even cancer. Fish oil also contains high levels of vitamin A, B3 and vitamin D.

Dandelion

If your dog suffers from digestive issues, dandelion may be a great herb to consider.

The dandelion flower may be used for its antioxidant properties and may improve the immune system. It is also high in lecithin.

Dandelion leaves are loaded with potassium. They also stimulate the appetite and help digestion along with kidney function. They are an ideal choice for dogs with chronic indigestion or those with gas.

Dandelion leaf also acts as a diuretic, making it useful in cases of arthritis, kidney stones, congestive heart failure and gallbladder disease. And best of all, dandelion leaf contains lots of potassium, which can be lost through urination. Dandelion leaf also stimulates the liver and promotes the elimination of waste material from the body.

Dandelion root is also quite useful and nutritional. The root is a liver tonic and helps to remove toxins from the body, via the kidneys. Signs of toxicity can include skin disease, dandruff and chronic constipation. Dandelion root can also treat gallstones and gallbladder inflammation.

Green lipped mussel

They contain a wide range of nutrients but their rare combination of omega 3 oils is what they are famous for. These oils, usually called green lipped mussel extract, are widely recognised as having an anti-inflammatory effect and are often recommended as a source of natural pain relief for dogs who suffer from arthritis.

Grains, Cereals

These are low-grade ingredients and are usually added to pet food as a source of fibre. Corn should be avoided due to dogs finding it hard to digest and may lead to food intolerance and allergies.

Brown rice/white rice

Brown rice comes in many forms and does contain beneficial nutrients. White rice should be avoided due to a rise in dogs being intolerant to it. White rice has no nutritional value.

Wheat

Again, this ingredient should be avoided and is usually found in lower grade dry dog food as its inexpensive and is ideal for forming biscuits and kibbles. Wheat should not be given to dogs who are wheat intolerant (also called Celiac), the gluten protein contained in the grain damages the lining of the small intestines and prevents it from absorbing parts of food that are important for staying healthy.

Alfalfa (Lucerne)

It's a medium quality ingredient and provides adequate nutrition. It is a natural source of iron, magnesium, vitamin A, C, E and several B vitamins and is a good source of fibre. It also contains a large amount of protein supplement which is not good for those dogs who need a low protein diet.

Carrots

Carrots are a good source of vitamin A which benefits the eyes to maintain healthy vision. They should be included in every diet and are a soluble fibre and full of natural anti-oxidants. Cooked carrots are easily digestible.

Chicory

Chicory is a good source of polysaccharide inulin and studies have shown they can have a beneficial effect on the guts 'good bacteria'. Inulin is quite sweet so it's added to pet food as a food flavour enhancer.

Derivatives of vegetable origins

This product is classed as low grade and can be from a wide range of ingredients. Manufacturers can change the product source from batch to batch. This can be particularly important if your dog is intolerant to certain ingredients. It is hard to identify what and where the product has come from.

Garlic

This is a high-quality ingredient with abundant beneficial nutrients. There is a lot of misleading information about garlic and owners are reluctant to use the product in their dog's diet. The fact is that small amounts of garlic can be extremely beneficial. Garlic can be an effective anti-fungal and anti-bacterial, it can help to eliminate intestinal worms and can act as a deterrent to skin parasites like fleas and ticks. Garlic can be very beneficial in lowering blood sugar in diabetics and can lower blood cholesterol. Some manufacturers use garlic to aid joint mobility problems. Garlic can be dangerous in high amounts. A 10kg dog would need to digest 2 whole bulbs for it to become toxic. 1 clove per 10kg of body weight per day is the recommended feeding guide. Please ensure you consult a nutritionist for advice.

Peas

Peas are classed as a quality ingredient with ample beneficial nutrients which are vitamin C, K and B1, manganese, fibre and folate.

Potatoes/potato starch/sugar beet and tapioca

These ingredients are OK but are used as a binding agent in grain free dry food. They all contain pure starch and nutritionists still doubt whether dogs can digest significant amounts of starch.

Sweet potato

Not a true potato but they are a very beneficial nutrient. They contain a lot more fibre and are a good source of vitamin A, C and B6. They have several minerals and are higher in sugar than the common potato. Recent studies have shown that sweet potato might actually be beneficial for diabetics since they can help stabilise blood sugar levels and lower insulin resistance. They're a high-quality carbohydrate source.

Vegetable protein extracts

Low grade and unsure what ingredients they may be referring to. Some nutritionists have speculated that vegetable protein extracts might also be a pseudonym for MSG (monosodium glutamate), This is the controversial food additive that some believe to be mildly addictive.

Yucca Extract

The extract is taken from the Yucca plant. It is said to naturally help the body remove toxins and aids digestion.

Borage oil/ Evening primrose oil

They are an excellent source of Gamm-linolenic acid (GLA) which has an anti-inflammatory effect and is often recommended in the natural treatment of arthritis. It is also used in the natural treatment of arthritis. It is also used to treat certain skin conditions.

Grape seed oil

This is a very beneficial ingredient and concerns lots of vital nutrients. Grape seed extract is a strong antioxidant that helps to support the immune system. It can also have an anti-inflammatory effect and is often recommended for dogs with an allergic-related skin condition. Unlike whole grapes, grape seed extract is not toxic to dogs.

Linseed/olive oil/sunflower oil

All these are good quality ingredient with beneficial nutrients. Linseed contains dietary fibre, lignin's, an abundance of micronutrients and omega 3 fatty acids. Olive oil benefits the coat and the heart and it contains vitamin E. Sunflower oil is pressed from sunflower seeds and is regarded as one of the healthier oils in dog foods. Its low in saturated fat and rich in the natural antioxidant vitamin E.

Psyllium

The husks of Psyllium seeds are usually added to dog foods as a source of soluble fibre which is important for maintaining digestive health.

Soya/soya bean proteins/soya meal

This is a controversial product which I recommend not using. They are high in protein and are often added to foods as a low-cost meat substitute. The proteins in soya are far less digestible and they are constantly linked to food intolerance and allergies.

Copper Sulphate

This is a controversial ingredient and I would recommend not using it. It is used as a copper supplement but in the EU, pure copper sulphate is classified as a 'harmful and dangerous to the environment as well as an irritant. Dogs need copper but they cannot make it themselves so it must be taken in through the diet. Although all dog foods naturally contain a certain amount of copper from the raw ingredient, additionally copper is routinely added as part of the multi mineral supplement found in almost all dog foods.

DL-methionine

Nutritionally adequate Methionine is an amino acid – a building block of protein. It is naturally found in a wide range of foods but is added to dog foods as it reduces the PH of the urine.

FOS

Fructo-oligo-saccharide is a nutritional supplement. It is becoming a more popular in dog foods due to its beneficial pre-biotic effect. It helps the growth of friendly bacteria.

L Carnitine

Carnitine is an amino acid (one of the building blocks of proteins) which is widely used with dogs with heart disorders and dogs on a weight loss programme.

Lysine

L-Lysine is a necessary building block for all proteins in a dog's body. It is an essential amino acid which means that it cannot be made by the dog's body so it has to be added to the dog's diet.

MOS

Mannan-oligo-saccharide is a nutritional supplement and is added to your dog's food for its beneficial pre-biotic effect. It aids the growth of friendly bacteria in the large intestines which promotes overall gastro-intestinal health. MOS is derived from the cell wall of yeasts.

MSM

Methyl-sulphonyl-methane is a natural derivate of pine bark. It is a treatment and prevention of osteoarthritis and other joint problems due to it anti-inflammatory effect.

Sodium Selenite

Sodium selenite can be controversial substance when it's used in a dog food recipe. That's because although the mineral is essential for normal cell function in all animals, selenium can be toxic in high doses.

Taurine

Taurine is an amino acid that can be found naturally in all sorts of food, especially seafood and meat. A number of studies have shown that taurine can help with the treatment of heart problems.

Artificial colourings

These are very controversial and I recommend trying to avoid. Studies has shown that these can cause behavioural problems, hyperactivity in our dogs. These can be shown on the ingredient list as sunset yellow, tartrazine, ponceau 4r, patent blue V and titanium dioxide. They can also be recognised as E numbers.

Artificial preservatives and antioxidants

These are added to the pet food to slow down spoilage. Preservatives used in pet foods are grouped into two general categories. Antimicrobials that block growth of bacteria, moulds or yeasts and antioxidants that slow the oxidation of fats and lipids that lead to the food going rancid. Most of these are artificially created. There are concerns over the damage which may be done to our pets.

Salt

Salt or sodium chloride as it is usually listed on the ingredient is added to pet food a flavour enhancer. Salt is a mineral and should not be added to food as it can already be found in raw ingredient. Dogs do enjoy the taste of salt and therefore manufacturers add it to the food to make it more appealing. This is very important if your dog suffers from heart problems or high blood pressure and should be avoided.

Oil and fats

Oils and fats either come from plants or animal sources. All dogs need some form of fat in their diet but it does not need to be added to food because oils and fat can be found naturally in all types of food. Natural oils and fats are better than low grade processed oils.

Sugars

Sugars are added to pet food because like humans, dogs love it. They are usually listed on the ingredient as sugar, caramel, syrup, sucrose etc. Sugars are sourced from corn, maize, wheat, sugar cane, sugar beet etc. High sugar diets have been linked to hyperactivity, hypoglycaemia, obesity and tooth decay. It should be avoided if possible.

Brewer's yeast

Yeast contains beneficial nutrients which are the best sources of natural B vitamins including B1 (thiamine), B2 (riboflavin), B3 (niacin), B5 (pantothenic acid), B6 (pyridoxine), B7 (biotin) and B9 (folic acid). These vitamins have a wide range of functions in dogs including supporting the nervous system, aiding the digestion, keeping the skin, hair, eyes, mouth, and liver healthy. Yeast is a good source of protein and contains essential amino acids.

Cellulose

Cellulose is a term used for low-grade dietary fibre. It is indigestible for dogs. It is usually found in light diets and cheaper diets to bulk out food with almost zero calories.

Charcoal

Charcoal absorbs excess gas and if often recommended for relieving wind and bloating in dogs. Active charcoal can come from wood, coconut shells, pet and bamboo.

Natural preservatives and antioxidants

All dried food contains preservatives. These are added to the food to stop the process which turns the fats rancid. Some manufacturers use highly controversial artificial preservatives but most are turning to more natural alternatives. The most common natural preservatives are Vitamin E (Tocopherols), vitamin C (ascorbic acid) and rosemary oil.

Phosphoric acid

This is a controversial ingredient. Phosphoric acid (E338) is a clear liquid that is added to food to stop the discolouration. It is usually added to cola drinks. Research and studies have shown that it can reduce bone density in humans but no studies have yet been made on animals.

Propylene glycol/ sodium Tripolyphosphate

Both are a synthetic compound. Propylene absorbs water. It is usually found in semi-moist food. It also has anti-bacterial and anti-fungal properties making it suitable as a preservative. Sodium tripolyphosphate (STPP or E451) is added to dog foods as a preservative and to help food retain its moisture. Both products should be avoided if possible.

BHA or BHT

Butylated hydroxy anisole or E320 and butylated hydroxytoluene or E321 are amongst the most common artificial antioxidants used in pet foods and are particularly worrying. A study and report at the University of Hamburg concluded that 'all published findings agree with the fact that BHA and BHT are tumour promoters' and the department of Health and Human studies in the US found that BHA consistently produces tumours in both rats and fish. The potential side-effects are not just physical with one study but finding a whole host of behavioural problems including increases aggression and a severe deficit in learning' is linked to BHA and BHT consumption in mice. Despite all the evidence both BHA and BHT are currently permitted in pet food (and human food) in both the US and in Europe.

Propyl Gallate (E310)

This is also an artificial preservative that is often used in conjunction with BHA and BHT. Again, it has been linked with tumours in mice.

Potassium Sorbate (E202) This can cause skin irritations and eye problems. It should be avoided if possible.

Unfortunately, you may not be able to avoid artificial preservatives and antioxidants. Over the years manufacturers have found ways to hide their usage of these ingredients.

Update: Ethoxyquin or E324 (which was widely used as an artificial antioxidant in pet foods and was thought to be responsible for allergic reactions, skin disease and behaviour problems) was suspended by the European Food Safety Authority in April 2017 on the basis that it caused damage to DNA and lead to cell mutation. As you can see this is only a suspension and not a ban. Ethoxyquin is still widely used outside of the EU.

When a pet food manufacturer adds preservatives to their products, they have to declare it on the label. Sometimes they don't list them on the ingredient but they list on the typical analysis. Some preservatives are listed as 'EU permitted antioxidants' as well.

Understanding veterinary lab tests

When your dog is unwell the vet will often ask for some routine tests to be conducted.

The complete blood count measures the number of cells of different types circulating in the bloodstream. There are three major types of blood cells in circulation; red blood cells (RBC), white blood cells (WBC), and platelets. Red blood cells are produced in the bone marrow, which is the soft centre of bones. RBCs pick up oxygen brought into the body by the lung's and bring oxygen to cells throughout the body. Red blood cells live in the blood stream for about 100 days although the actual time varies with the type of animal. Old red blood cells are removed from the blood stream by the spleen and liver. Red blood cell numbers can be decreased (anaemia) if they are not produced in adequate numbers by the bone marrow, if their life span is shortened (a condition called haemolysis), or if they are lost due to bleeding. Increased red blood cell numbers is called polycythaemia and is usually due to concentration of the blood due to dehydration.

The complete blood count also includes a measure of haemoglobin, which is the actual substance in the red blood cell that carries oxygen.

There are several types of white blood cells in blood, including neutrophils (PMNs), lymphocytes, monocytes, eosinophils and basophils. Lymphocytes are produced in lymph nodes throughout the body. The other white blood cell types are produced in the bone marrow along with the red blood cells and platelets. The majority of white blood cells in circulation are neutrophils, which help the animal fight infections. Neutrophils can be decreased in pets with bone marrow disease, in some viral diseases, and in some pets receiving cancer chemotherapy drugs. Neutrophils are increased in pets with inflammation or infection of any part of the body and in pets receiving prednisone or other cortisone-type drugs. Lymphocytes also help fight infection and produce antibodies against infectious agents (viruses, bacteria, etc.). Lymphocytes may be increased in puppies and kittens with an infection, they can be decreased in pets who are severely stressed, and lymphocytes might be lost in some types of diarrhoea. Certain drugs, such as prednisone (a cortisone-type drug) will decrease the number of lymphocytes in the blood stream.

Monocytes may be increased in pets with chronic infections. Eosinophils and basophils are increased in pets with allergic diseases, or parasitic infections (worms, fleas, etc.).

Platelets are produced in the bone marrow and are involved in the process of making a blood clot. Platelets live a few weeks and are constantly being produced by the bone marrow. Low platelet counts occur if the bone marrow is damaged and doesn't produce them, or if the platelets are destroyed at a faster rate than normal. The two primary causes of platelet destruction are immune-mediated destruction (ITP or IMT) and DIC (disseminated intravascular coagulation). Immune-mediated thrombocytopenia happens when the animal's immune system destroys platelets. DIC is a complex problem in which blood clots form in the body using the platelets faster than the bone marrow can produce new ones. Animals with a low platelet count bruise easily and may have blood in their urine or stool.

Packed cell volume (PCV) (called haematocrit) is another measure of red blood cells. A small amount of blood is placed in a tiny glass tube and spun in a centrifuge. The blood cells pack to the bottom of the tube and the fluid floats on top. The PCV is the percent of blood, that is cells, compared to the total volume of blood. In normal dogs and cats, 40-50% of the blood is made up of blood cells and the remainder is fluid.

Blood and urine tests are performed to get an initial overview of the health, and sometimes the function, of body organs. Some blood tests are very specific for a single organ, whereas other tests are affected by several organs. Blood tests are often performed as a biochemistry profile, or chemistry panel, which is a collection of blood tests to screen several organs at one time. The makeup of a biochemical profile varies with the laboratory in which it is performed. Following are some of the more commonly performed chemical tests:

Albumin is a small protein produced by the liver. Albumin acts as a sponge to hold water in the blood vessels. When blood albumin is decreased, the pressure created by the heart forcing blood through the blood vessels causes fluid to leak out of the blood vessels and accumulate in body cavities such as the abdominal cavity or in tissues as oedema. Albumin is decreased if the liver is damaged and cannot produce an adequate amount of albumin or if albumin is lost through damaged intestine or in the urine due to kidney disease. The only cause of increased albumin is dehydration.

Alkaline phosphatase originates from many tissues in the body. When alkaline phosphatase is increased in the bloodstream of a dog the most common causes are liver disease, bone disease or increased blood cortisol either because prednisone or similar drug is being given to the pet or because the animal has Cushing's disease (hypoadrenocorticism). In cats, the most common causes of increased alkaline phosphatase are liver and bone disease.

ALT is an enzyme produced by liver cells. Liver damage causes ALT to increase in the bloodstream. ALT elevation does not provide information as to whether the liver disease is reversible or not.

Amylase is an enzyme produced by the pancreas and the intestinal tract. Amylase helps the body breakdown sugars. Amylase may be increased in the blood in animals with inflammation (pancreatitis) or cancer of the pancreas. Sometimes pancreatitis is difficult to diagnose and some dogs and cats with pancreatitis will have normal amounts of amylase in the blood. Lipase is another pancreatic enzyme which is responsible for the breakdown of fats and which may be increased in patients with pancreatic inflammation or cancer.

Bile acids are produced by the liver and are involved in fat breakdown. A bile acid test is used to evaluate the function of the liver and the blood flow to the liver. Patients with abnormal blood flow to the liver, a condition known as portosystemic shunt will have abnormal levels of bile acids. The bile acid test measures a fasting blood sample and a blood sample two hour after eating.

Bilirubin is produced by the liver from old red blood cells. Bilirubin is further broken down and eliminated in both the urine and stool. Bilirubin is increased in the blood in patients with some types of liver disease, gallbladder disease or in patients who are destroying the red blood cells at a faster than normal rate (haemolysis). Large amounts of bilirubin in the bloodstream will give a yellow colour to non-furred parts of the body, which is called icterus or jaundice. Icterus is most easily recognized in the tissues around the eye, inside the ears and on the gums.

BUN (blood urea nitrogen) is influenced by the liver, kidneys, and by dehydration. Blood urea nitrogen is a waste product produced by the liver from proteins from the diet and is eliminated from the body by the kidneys. A low BUN can be seen with liver disease and an increased BUN is seen in pets with kidney disease. The kidneys must be damaged to the point that 75% of the kidneys are non-functional before BUN will increase. Pets that are severely dehydrated will have an increased BUN as the kidneys of a dehydrated patient don't get a normal amount of blood presented to them, so the waste products do not get to the kidneys to be eliminated.

Calcium in the bloodstream originates from the bones. The body has hormones, which cause bone to release calcium into the blood and to remove calcium from the blood and place it back into bone. Abnormally high calcium in the blood occurs much more commonly than low calcium. High blood calcium is most commonly associated with cancer. Less common causes of elevated calcium are chronic kidney failure, primary hyperparathyroidism which is over-function of the parathyroid gland, poisoning with certain types of rodent bait and bone disease.

Low blood calcium may occur in dogs and cats just before giving birth or while they are nursing their young. This is called eclampsia and occurs more commonly in small breed dogs. Eclampsia causes the animal to have rigid muscles which is called tetany. Another cause of low blood calcium is malfunction of the parathyroid glands which produce a hormone (PTH) that controls blood calcium levels. Animals poisoned with antifreeze may have a very low blood calcium.

Cholesterol is a form of fat. Cholesterol can be increased in the bloodstream for many reasons in dogs. It is much less common for cats to have increased cholesterol. Some of the diseases that cause elevated cholesterol are hypothyroidism, Cushing's disease, diabetes and kidney diseases that cause protein to be lost in the urine. High cholesterol does not predispose dogs and cats to heart and blood vessel disease as it does in people.

Creatinine is a waste product that originates from muscles and is eliminated from the body by the kidneys. An elevation of creatinine is due to kidney disease or dehydration. Both creatinine and BUN increase in the bloodstream at the same time in patients with kidney disease.

Creatinine kinase (CK) is released into the blood from damaged muscle. Elevation of creatinine kinase therefore suggests damage to muscle including heart muscle.

Glucose is blood sugar. Glucose is increased in dogs and cats with diabetes mellitus. It may be mildly increased in dogs with Cushing's disease. Glucose can temporarily increase in the blood if the dog or cat is excited by having a blood sample drawn. This is especially true of cats. A quick test to determine whether a glucose elevation is transient or permanent is to look at the urine. If the glucose is chronically elevated there will be an increased amount of glucose in the urine as well.
Low blood sugar occurs less commonly and can be a sign of pancreatic cancer or overwhelming infection (sepsis). Low blood sugar can cause depression or seizures. Low blood sugar can be seen if the blood sample is improperly handled. Red blood cells will use glucose so typically red blood cells are removed from the blood sample and the clear part of the blood (plasma or serum), is used for analysis.

Phosphorus in the bloodstream originates from bones and is controlled by the same hormone, PTH (parathyroid hormone) which controls blood calcium. Phosphorus is increased in the bloodstream in patients with chronic kidney disease. Like BUN and creatinine, phosphorus increases in these patients when about 75 percent of both kidneys is damaged.

Potassium is increased in the bloodstream in the pet with acute kidney failure such as kidney failure caused by antifreeze poisoning, in dogs with Addison's disease and in animals with a ruptured or obstructed bladder.

Potassium is lost from the body in vomit, diarrhoea and urine. Pets that are not eating may have a low blood potassium. Low blood potassium can cause the pet to feel weak. Cats with low potassium may develop painful muscles.

Sodium may be slightly increased in the blood if the patient is dehydrated although many dehydrated dogs and cats have a normal blood sodium. Low blood sodium is most commonly seen with Addison's disease (hypoadrenocorticism).

Total protein includes albumin and larger proteins called globulins. Included in the globulins are antibodies which are protein molecules. Total protein can be increased if the dog or cat is dehydrated or if the pet's immune system is being stimulated to produce large amounts of antibody. Total protein is decreased in the same situations which reduce albumin or if the pet has an abnormal immune system and cannot produce antibodies.

Urinalysis: A urine sample can provide information about several organ systems. The concentration, colour, clarity and microscopic examination of the urine sample can provide diagnostic information.

Urine may be obtained by catching a sample during normal urination, by passing a catheter into the bladder or by placing a small needle through the body wall into the bladder, a procedure called cystocentesis. Depending upon why the urine sample is being collected, one collection method may be preferred over another. Enquire at the time you make an appointment for veterinary care if a urine sample may be collected. Preventing your pet from urinating prior to the appointment will assure that your pet's bladder will contain urine for sampling.

Complete Blood Count (CBC)

This is the most common blood test performed on pets and people. A CBC gives information on hydration status, anaemia, infection, the blood's clotting ability, and the ability of the immune system to respond. This test is essential for pets with fevers, vomiting, diarrhoea, weakness, pale gums, or loss of appetite. If your pet needs surgery, a CBC can detect some bleeding disorders or other unseen abnormalities.

Red Cell Count measures the total number of red blood cells per volume of blood. It is used in detecting anaemia and other disorders of red blood cells. MCV (Mean Cell Volume) measures the volume of the individual red blood cell.

- **Haemoglobin** is the oxygen-carrying pigment of red blood cells. **MCHC** and **MCH** (mean corpuscular haemoglobin concentration and mean corpuscular haemoglobin) are all measures of haemoglobin and used in differentiating some anaemias.

- **PCV** (packed Cell Volume or haematocrit) measures the percentage of red blood cells to detect anaemia and dehydration.

White Cell Count (white blood cell count) measures the body's immune cells. Increases or decreases may indicate certain diseases, infections or inflammation.

- **Neutrophils, lymphocytes** and **monocytes** are specific types of white blood cells. Disturbances of these may indicate infection, stress, cancer, hormonal imbalances and other conditions.

- **Eosinophils** are a specific type of white blood cell that may indicate allergic or parasitic conditions.

Platelet count measures cells that help to form blood clots.

Reticulocytes are immature red blood cells. High levels indicate rebuilding of red blood cell numbers.

Blood chemistries

These common blood serum tests evaluate organ function, electrolyte status, hormone levels and more. They are important in evaluating older pets, pets with vomiting, diarrhoea or toxin exposure, pets receiving long-term medications and health before anaesthesia.

- **Na** (sodium) is an electrolyte lost with vomiting, diarrhoea, kidney disease and Addison's disease. This test helps indicate hydration status.

- **K** (potassium) is an electrolyte lost with vomiting, diarrhoea or excessive urination. Increased levels may indicate kidney failure, Addison's disease, dehydration or urethral obstruction. High levels can lead to a heart attack.

- **Cl** (chloride) is an electrolyte often lost with vomiting and Addison's disease. Elevations often indicate dehydration.

- **Bicarb** is an indication of acid / base balance and can be changed with vomiting and other conditions.

- **BUN** (blood urea nitrogen) indicates kidney function. An increased level in the blood is called azotaemia and can be caused by kidney, liver, heart disease, urethral obstruction, shock and dehydration.

- **CREA** (creatinine) reveals kidney function. This test helps distinguish between kidney and non-kidney causes of elevated BUN

- **Ca** (calcium) deviations can indicate a variety of diseases. Tumours, hyperparathyroidism, kidney disease and low albumin are just a few of the conditions that alter serum calcium.

- **PHOS** (phosphorus) elevations are often associated with kidney disease, hyperthyroidism and bleeding disorders.

- **AMYL** (amylase) elevation may indicate pancreatitis or kidney disease.

- **LIP** (lipase) is an enzyme that may indicate pancreatitis.

- **TP** (total protein) indicates hydration status and provides additional information about the liver, kidneys and infectious diseases.

- **ALB** (albumin) is a serum protein that helps evaluate hydration, haemorrhage, intestinal, liver, and kidney disease.

- **GLOB** (globulin) is a blood protein that often increases with chronic inflammation and certain disease states, including some cancers.

- **TBIL** (total bilirubin) elevations may indicate liver or haemolytic disease. This test helps identify bile duct problems and certain types of anaemia.

- **ALKP** (alkaline phosphatase) elevations may indicate liver damage, Cushing's disease or active bone growth in young pets. This test is especially significant in cats.

- **ALT** (alanine aminotransferase) is a sensitive indicator of active liver damage but doesn't indicate the cause.

- **GGT** (gamma glutamyl transferase) is an enzyme that indicates liver disease or corticosteroid excess.

- **AST** (aspartate aminotransferase) increase may indicate liver, heart or skeletal muscle damage.

- **CK** (Creatine Kinase) is an enzyme that indicates muscle damage.

- **LDH** (Lactic Dehydrogenase) is an enzyme that can be elevated in muscle, heart and liver disease.

- **CHOL** (cholesterol) is used to aid in the diagnosis of hypothyroidism, liver disease, Cushing's disease and diabetes mellitus.

- **GLU** (glucose) is a blood sugar. Elevated levels may indicate diabetes mellitus. Low levels can cause collapse, seizures or coma.

- **Cortisol** is a hormone that is measured in tests for Cushing's disease (the low-dose dexamethasone suppression test) and Addison's disease (ACTH stimulation test)

- **T4** (thyroxine) is a thyroid hormone. Decreased levels often signal hypothyroidism in dogs, while high levels may indicate hyperthyroidism in cats.

Results for trial Research

The trial supplement contained: Live yeast, prebiotic, probiotic, SC1-1077, chicory inulin, ground chickweed, milled linseed. Cereal was added to those dogs who could tolerate gluten.

The Flower Remedy, labelled CECS Flower Remedy was based on Dr Bach's research. The ingredient used was Star of Bethlehem, Impatiens, Mimulus, Cherry plum, Rock rose.

Both products are available to buy (www.handsandpaws.co.uk) The CECS supplement is now Gluten free and is called Natural Restore Supplement.

14 dogs took part over a period of 12 months (Nov 2014 to Oct 2015)

Trial Supplement
CECS Flower remedies

14 dogs affected with CECS
4 Colitis sufferers

14/14   No reports of dogs refusing to eat food with supplement in.
11/14   Dogs drank water with liquid supplement in without any problems.
3/14   Refused to drink water with drops added.
8/14   Dogs appetites increased
12/14   Owners saw a significant change in their dog's health and personality within 2 to 5 days of being on the supplement and drops.
12/14   Owners reported an improvement in fur and skin condition as well as black wet nose

8/14 Owners reported their dog as less stressed, more settled and less aggressive towards other dogs
7/14 Owners reported weight increase but at a healthy rate.
5/14 Dog's maintained their weight
2/14 Reported dogs had lost weight but they were overweight to begin with
8/14 Reported normal poo's
3/14 Reported firmer poo's
1/14 Reported constipation (reduced dosage to correct)
2/14 Reported that poo's had improved
2/14 Reported anal gland problem had disappeared since being on the supplement
4/14 Reported their dog's breath had improved and they had less wind
12/14 No reports of yellow or white bile regurgitation.
1/14 Reported of vomiting food once while being on the trial
1/14 Vomited bile with grass
8/14 Reported less grass eating while exercising
6/14 N/A
7/14 Reported no grumbly or noisy tummies   7/14 N/A

Effect the supplement had on non-related allergies not associated with CECS or Colitis.

2/14 Dogs had itchy paws before the supplement. All problems now resolved within 2 weeks of taking supplements.
2/14 Dogs suffered with ear mites before the trial have now reported no problems with ears.
1/14 Dog suffered with eczema on inside hind leg and on the belly have said 2 weeks after using the supplement the condition had cleared up and now she has stopped the steroids and her dog is happy again.

2/14 Colitis dogs who were intolerant to gluten have now been placed on a pet food which has gluten in and they can now tolerate it without any adverse effect.
1/14 CECS dogs who were intolerant to gluten can now tolerate it.

CECS results

6/8   Owners reported no CECS episodes over a period of 3 months.
1/8   One owner whose dog was having 2 episodes a day has not had one since starting the supplement 6 weeks ago.
2/8   Reported 3 episodes but these were a lot less aggressive and were shorter

Colitis results
3 /4   Reported no colitis while being on the supplement
1 /4   Reported a colitis bout. Did admit her dog had eaten a Farley's rusk the day before which may have affected the result.
4/4   Reported overall health had improved over the 3-month period.

Overall findings: The supplement seems to help and aid a number of digestive illnesses as well as skin problems resulting from allergies. The research shows that the supplement can in, most situations, manage and reduce the number of CECS episodes. No matter what the trigger is for these episodes the supplement works by controlling what nutrients vitamins, minerals, amino acids and enzymes are needed by the body by way of the gut, the liver, the kidneys and pancreas. After this process they are evenly distributed then at a normal rate of which the digestive system can deal with. It may help to remove toxins as well as stabilise the stomach acids and reduce the amount of white or yellow bile being produced It also lines the gut wall and acts as a barrier against harmful bacteria. All round it improves general health, skin and coat condition and will result in less tummy noises and can help aid the digestion process so the gut has less chance to go into cramp or feel uncomfortable for your dog.

What does the future hold for the Border Terrier?

I fear for the breeds future and what may become of it in 20 years' time. My research has shown that there is a lot of controversy surrounding illnesses and conditions which are associated with the breed. There seems to be a lack of knowledge whether it's with the breeders, veterinary practices, the show world and the pet owner. When asking owners who have experienced CECS if they would consider getting another border terrier quite a few have said no due to the stress of seeing their dog suffering from this condition. I have found that some breeders of Border terriers have now stopped due to problems they are encountering with past litters, even though both parents may not show signs of any problems.

Education and awareness is the key to managing this condition until researchers find a true cause to this illness. CECS is not life threatening and does not cause any impediment to the dog's life. With diet management, reduction of chemicals and possible triggers there is no reason why a CECS dog cannot live a long and happy life.

Summary for management of CECS

- Choose a Gluten free diet
- A food which is low in vegetable or plant protein but high in meat protein
- Filter or distilled water
- Remove Rawhide chews
- Only feed natural treats (no colourings, preservatives, salts or sugars)
- Remove possible triggers
- Aid supplements to help with digestion
- Dental health is a must. Scaling teeth and removing any bad teeth. Brush daily
- Use herbal remedies to help your dog relax in stressful situations
- Do not use chemical wormers or flea products
- Only have annual boosters if really necessary (Antibody test)
- If possible use natural food or a homecooked diet
- Remove all air refreshers, plug in's etc
- Replace any metal bowls with porcelain ones
- Try to avoid chemical Flea, tick and worming treatments

- Use low fat products

- Avoid foods with large amounts of fillers

Research and tests are still ongoing for the reason for this illness and hopefully a way to treat the condition.

I hope this book has given you a better understanding and insight into CECS and a chance for owners to manage the condition the best possible way. The contents of this book are based on my studying and personal research. Always seek help and advice from your vet.

Further information

http://www.handsandpaws.co.uk

Facebook: Canine Epileptoid Cramping Syndrome group

Animal Health Trust: http://www.aht.org.uk/

The Author: handsandpaws@hotmail.com

Supplements & flower remedies
http://www.handsandpaws.co.uk

ISBN 978-1-5272-2275-5